Care of the Difficult Patient

Developed collaboratively by a doctor and nurse, this is the first text to deal specifically with nursing difficult patients. Whether problems stem from mental distress and ill health, historic substance abuse, demanding family members or abusive behaviour, difficult patients place extra demands on nurses both professionally and personally. Caring for difficult patients requires technical and interpersonal skills, and the ability to exercise power and set limits.

This text presents invaluable practical recommendations, well founded in experience and supported by relevant literature, for nurses coping with challenging, real world situations. Covering pertinent issues such as manipulative and sexually inappropriate behaviour, anger and violence, delirium, setting limits, death and dying, difficult doctors, psychiatric diagnoses, the text includes learning points, further reading, case studies and dialogue examples to highlight good (and bad) practice. Ideal for pre- and post-registration nurses, this reference provides concrete direction on the management of difficult patients.

Peter J. Manos is a consultation-liaison psychiatrist in a general hospital and is on the clinical faculty at the University of Washington School of Medicine.
Joan Braun has been a medical/surgical nurse and nurse educator for thirty-seven years.

Care of the Difficult Patient

A Nurse's Guide

Peter J. Manos and Joan Braun

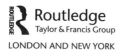
Routledge
Taylor & Francis Group

LONDON AND NEW YORK

First published 2006
by Routledge
2 Park Square, Milton Park, Abingdon, OX14 4RN

Simultaneously published in the USA and Canada
by Routledge
270 Madison Ave, New York, NY 10016

Reprinted 2006

Routledge is an imprint of the Taylor & Francis Group, an informa business

© 2006 Peter J. Manos and Joan Braun

Typeset in Sabon by
Keystroke, Jacaranda Lodge, Wolverhampton
Printed and bound in Great Britain by
TJ International Ltd, Padstow, Cornwall

British Library Cataloguing in Publication Data
A catalogue record for this book is available from the British Library

Library of Congress Cataloging in Publication Data
A catalog record for this book has been requested

ISBN10: 0–415–35823–X   ISBN13: 9–78–0–415–35823–1 (hbk)
ISBN10: 0–415–35824–8   ISBN13: 9–78–0–415–35824–8 (pbk)

Contents

List of tables and figure

Figure

Acknowledgments

The following people have provided us with concrete support in the form of written comments on the manuscript, supportive listening and encouragement, editorial guidance, or in ways it is prudent to leave unmentioned (a little mystery never hurt an acknowledgment page). We thank them. Hundreds of other colleagues helped teach us this subject matter over the past 30 years. We are sorry we are unable to thank them all by name.

J. H. Atkinson, M.D., Teresa Anderson, R.N., Hillis Backman, R.N., Carol Blainey, R.N. M.N., C.D.E., Penny Ford Carleton, R.N., M.S., M.P.A., Kris Cimino, R.N., Mary E. Clark, Ph.D., Anne Cunha, R.N., Janis Cunningham, R.R.T., Suzanne Eilers, R.N., Kappy Finstuen, R.N., B.D.N., O.C.N., Amber Frymier, R.N., Nina Gurr, R.N., Bertha Hanson, R.N., Mary Hansen, R.N., Judy Hoeffer, R.N., Eileen Hurlbert, R.N., Connie Hirnle, R.N., M.N., Gale Hurley, R.N., Richard Kozarek, M.D., Susan Schweinsburg Long, M.S.L., A.H.I.P, Carole Love, R.N., Chen-chen Lee, R.N., Maja Quist-McLeary, R.N., Amy Myoraku, R.N., Sheila McNamara, R.N., Sandy Maloof, R.N., Jennifer Moen, R.N., Art Morrill, R.N., Elaine Muecklisch, R.N., Cathy Nunnely, R.N., Clydia Pappenfus, R.N., Cynthia Pompei, R.N., Christina Patopea, R.N., Mary Alice Power, R.N., Ann R. Quealy, R.N., M.S.N., Anne Reiner, R.N., Dave Strauss, C.F.A., Julie Smith, B.A., Paula Smith, R.N., Alice Shreve, R.N., Skye Stott, R.N., Brooke Stevens, R.N., Stephanie Shen, Becky Stewart, R.N., M.S.N., Linda Trafton, P.T., William Traverso, M.D., Ellie Yuen, R.N.

We thank Karen Bowler for her astute interest in publishing the manuscript and Claire Gauler for her good-humored responsiveness to questions about its preparation. We are grateful for the sincere interest and help in this project of our production editor, Fiona Wade, and marketing executive, Hannah Qualtrough.

To our spouses, Dr. Ingrid Dinter and Mr. Steve Braun, we especially express our gratitude.

Research for this book was greatly assisted by Virginia Mason Medical Library.

Virginia Mason Medical Center continues to provide the authors a felicitous setting for continued collaboration in the care of patients.

Introduction

This book grew from our collaboration together for over twenty-one years as med/surg staff nurse and consultation-liaison psychiatrist on the wards of a general medical hospital. Because literally hundreds of nurses we have worked with over the years have benefited from the ideas we present here, we are confident that what we have to say is useful and can benefit even more clinical nurses and their patients.

Nurses working in the general hospital today are being asked to help stabilize patients as quickly as possible not only for the patients' benefit, but to shorten their length of stay. Insurance companies are unwilling to pay for hospital days if they believe them medically unnecessary. This focus on shortening average length of stay has its good and bad sides, which can be debated. One thing is certain, however: demands are increasing on nurses to be maximally efficient. Maximally efficient, yes, but with fewer nurses per patient. Complicating matters is that today's in-patients are much sicker than were yesteryears', yet communication and continuity of care is harder because of more transient staffs: per diem and traveling nurses; and rapid turnover of unlicensed staff.

In this setting, difficult patients present a dilemma not only for their primary nurses but also for the other nurses on the ward, and for nurse supervisors and administrators. A difficult patient may not only have an unnecessarily long hospital stay but disrupt the entire ward routine as well. A nurse skilled in caring for such a patient is an asset to everyone concerned but it often takes years to develop the necessary skills. Skill development can be accelerated. We envision this book being used by practicing nurses, perhaps first as a guide for a continuing education course or senior level nursing school course. We believe that nurse supervisors will use it to help their colleagues care for difficult patients. We have, however, written a book that is enjoyable to read and believe that you, the nurse reading this introduction, may simply wish to have it for your own reference whatever your specific use of it may be. By reading this book, you will be better able to exercise your power to effectively care for difficult patients.

The attributes that make a patient difficult reside not within the patient but within the relationship with the nurse. The patient is viewed by nurses as difficult when one or more of the following apply: behavior conflicts with the expected patient role; personality or behavior conflict with the nurse's values; or the patient appears to challenge the nurses' control (MacDonald 2003). We define the difficult patient as one whose behavior is an obstacle to the provision of good nursing care.

The committed, involved stance of caring is central to nursing practice, but as Benner (1984) notes there are different kinds of caring in different contexts. Nor does caring preclude the nurse's exercise of power: on the contrary, it demands it. Caring for difficult patients involves technical and interpersonal skills, but also draws on the nurse's sense of self and ability to exercise power and set limits. Since the exercise of power and setting of limits is, in some sense, central to the care of difficult patients we dedicate separate chapters to the nurse's authority, to the feelings evoked in nurses by difficult patients, and to limit setting.

Because some nurses may feel that the firm setting of limits is unnecessarily harsh, we wish to emphasize now at the onset, that underlying everything we have to say about setting limits with difficult patients is our assumption that the nurse will best be able to attend to the medical, nursing, and personal needs of the difficult patient, i.e., best be able *care* for the difficult patient, by using the approaches we suggest. Some of these patients are referred to in the literature as "hateful patients" because of the unpleasant emotions they elicit in their caregivers, but we hope, perhaps too idealistically, that given an effective approach to managing them, nurses will find none of them "hateful" (Groves 1978).

The lack of love in infancy and childhood of many patients leads to problematic behavior later in life. Other patients are difficult because they are delirious, drug or alcohol dependent, frightened, angry, or needy. On the other hand, who is to say how you, the reader, or we the writers, would behave were we hospitalized for months with necrotizing pancreatitis or acute lymphocytic leukemia. The threats of serious illness – pain, nausea, dyspnea, disability, impoverishment, dependence, and death – could transform any of us into a difficult patient.

In this book, we do not delve into psychological explanations of why people behave the way they do. We do not provide developmental histories. We describe behaviors and what to do about them. Our approach is practical, not theoretical.

The novice and advanced beginner will find here concrete direction on the management of difficult patients, advice that may spare both patient and nurse considerable future frustration. The proficient and expert nurse, we hope, will find affirmation of her or his hard earned experience as well as a fresh look at psychotropic and analgesic medications, assessment, and nurse–nurse and nurse–doctor communication.

Though the subject of this book is serious, it need not be dreary. We have allowed ourselves to be whimsical, imagining, for example, the tirade of a frustrated nurse telling a delirious and paranoid patient that she will not call a cab for him to go home one day after his hip surgery. Even Hedwig, the owl, and Hagrid, the half giant, appear.

Although most nurses are women, more and more men are entering the profession. Principally we refer to the nurse as "she", less frequently as "he".

A respiratory therapist who took our course on the care of the difficult patient told us that the book should also be read by respiratory therapists, occupational therapists, speech therapists, and case managers. We hope it will be.

We begin with a chapter on mental status testing because patients can't be cared for, their problems and problematic behavior managed, until mood and cognition are assessed. We include many cases histories.

Limit setting, a cornerstone for the management of many difficult patients, is reviewed in Chapter 5.

This book was written to be read, not just referred to in times of crisis. We believe you will enjoy it.

Joan Braun, R.N.
Peter J. Manos, M.D.

Bibliography

Benner PE. 1984 *From Novice to Expert: Excellence and Power in Clinical Nursing Practice*. Menlo Park, Calif.: Addison-Wesley Pub. Co., Nursing Division.

MacDonald M. 2003 Seeing the cage: stigma and its potential to inform the concept of the difficult patient. *Clinical Nurse Specialist*. 17(6):305–10; quiz 311–12, Nov.

Groves JE. 1978 Taking care of the hateful patient. *The New England Journal of Medicine*. 298:883–7.

Chapter 1

Mental status assessment

Pam Green, R.N., works on an oncology unit, having graduated from nursing school a year and a half ago. Her new patient, Mr. Allen Johnson, a high school English teacher who worked until a week prior to admission, has just been admitted for chemotherapy of his newly diagnosed, inoperable pancreatic cancer. He is terse, formal, and remote. His wife provides Pam with most of the intake history.

The next day he has not gotten up to eat breakfast. Pam enters the room.

"Good morning, Mr. Johnson."

Initially lying on his left side facing the door, he turns away from her and pulls the covers over his head.

"Mr. Johnson, may I help you with something?"

"No, I'm fine."

"You didn't eat any breakfast."

"I'm fine."

"I'd just like to get your blood pressure and temperature."

Earlier he had refused to let the nursing assistant get his vital signs. Now, reluctantly, he allows it.

"Try to have some breakfast, Mr. Johnson."

Sadly recalling the association between pancreatic cancer and depression, she leaves the room, intending to return shortly.

Later, the blanket removed from his head, Mr. Johnson is picking at the sheets and grimacing.

"Mr. Johnson, what's wrong?"

"Don't give me that innocent bullshit. You know what's wrong, alright."

"Are you in pain?"

"Don't come near me, do you understand?"

Because she doesn't know what's going on, Pam is unsure what to do next, but she heeds the fear she feels and does not approach any closer.

"I'm going to get some morphine. I'll be right back."

At the narcotics cart, she sees her respected colleague, Susan Eiman, R.N., and explains her consternation.

"I don't know how much morphine to give. He had a lot last night but I think he wants more."

"Did you examine him?" asks Susan.

"He won't let me."

"What does he tell you?"

"Not much."

On Susan's recommendation, they look at the night shift nursing notes. Mr. Johnson was quiet most of the night but he's also described as "forgetful". He had a low-grade fever. Together they return to his room. Just inside the doorway, Susan stops.

"Mr. Johnson, my name is Susan. I'm a nurse here at City Hospital. I'm coming in for a minute to talk."

She then slowly walks around the bed to face the patient, pulls up a chair four feet away from him, and sits down. The sheets and blankets are twisted and in disarray. There is a urine stain on the sheet. She says nothing for a whole minute, which feels like ten minutes to Pam. Finally Susan speaks.

"What's on your mind, Mr. Johnson?"

"Leave me alone."

"You're in the hospital and we're your nurses here. We want to help you. Please tell us what's bothering you."

No response.

"Mr. Johnson, please tell us what's bothering you."

No response.

"Did anything unusual or frightening happen last night?"

"Just the wedding. How can you so-called nurses have a wedding when there are people dying in here?"

After they leave the room, Susan explains that Mr. Johnson is delirious and gets an order for some IV haloperidol. She withholds the opioids that might have been contributing to the delirium, and calls the intern to express concern that the patient's fever might be due to pneumonia or a urinary tract infection and which also might be contributing to the delirium.

Susan Eiman, R.N., an expert clinician, suspects from the onset that this is not a case of depression or anger. Checking the night notes she finds that the patient is described as "forgetful". She persists in asking questions, even when put off by the patient. The patient responds strangely. His judgment appears impaired. He finally expresses his delusions and hallucinations about the nurses having a wedding outside his room. Aided by her experience, Ms. Eiman has assessed his mental status, though she did not follow a fixed set of questions to do so. Because she is a nurse, just sitting at the bedside and looking at the patient, she is doing an assessment. She might not even be able to voice all the elements of her observations. In this chapter, we offer you an outline of a mental status examination, and some specific questions that you may find useful.

Parts of a mental status examination

Evaluation of any problematic behavior demands at least some attempt to assess the patient's mental status. A mnemonic will help you recall the outline of a mental status examination that can help you organize your thinking: A Beast Prom (or A Beast Romp, if you like) (Table 1).

Table 1 A mnemonic for the parts of a mental status examination

Appearance

Behavior

Emotion (mood)

Affect

Speech

Thoughts (delusional, suicidal, homicidal, violent)

Perception (hallucinations)

Reasoning (including judgment and insight)

Orientation

Memory

Appearance

Facial expression may be tense, worried, sad, happy, sneering, ecstatic, pained, angry, laughing, suspicious.

You may wish to describe appearance only at your initial evaluation or if a change occurs. Note unique facial features, tattoos, jewelry, body piercing, grooming, hygiene, posture, and the presence of IV lines, drains, catheters, monitors, bandages, and restraints.

Appearance may give diagnostic clues:[1] poor fingernail hygiene is often associated with dementia because demented patients overlook grooming. An excessive display of masculine symbols may give clues to the diagnosis of antisocial personality disorder: heavy chains, a knife worn on the belt, the tattoo "born to lose" on the deltoid or "H A T E" on the knuckles of one hand, "L O V E" on the knuckles of the other, a heavy belt buckle, and so forth.

Although generally part of the physical examination, you should consider pupil size as part of your evaluation. Opioid intoxication is often associated with small pupils but pupils tend to become smaller as people age (Buckley *et al.* 1987; Pickworth *et al.* 1989; Hennelly *et al.* 1998).

Anxiety is often associated with large pupils (Lader 1983). In the general hospital though, interpretation of pupillary size is complicated because other medications may affect them. Recall, too, that people's pupillary size diminishes with age.

Behavior

Is the patient drowsy, alert, restless, agitated?

Agitation is purposeless motor activity: pacing, picking at the air or at bedclothes and sheets, constantly shifting position in bed, or repeatedly sitting and then standing. It is usually associated with anxiety, that is, fear without an object of fear. Agitation is worrisome. It should be documented and evaluated. Agitation may be caused by anger, fear, delirium, pain, and physiological deterioration – new fever, new pneumonia, new hemorrhage, etc. Is the patient experiencing drug withdrawal? Is the patient experiencing an acute dystonia or other extrapyramidal side effects such as akathisia?[2] (Ferrando and Eisendrath 1991).

On the other hand, the patient may simply lie in bed, unmoving, minimally responsive. It is commonly assumed that such a patient is depressed; consider, however, over-sedation, pain, nausea, dyspnea, delirium, hypotension, electrolyte imbalance, etc.

The following adjectives also describe behavior: irritable, sullen, resentful, indifferent, friendly, dramatic, impulsive, evasive, cooperative, flirtatious, etc. Strong descriptions, however, cannot depend on adjectives. Verbs and nouns are more precise and better understood. A brief, concrete, written description of your patient's behavior may be helpful to the entire staff. "Ate all her breakfast. Slept well. Up and about without difficulty. Talked on the phone and laughed." If the patient is concurrently complaining of intolerable pain, something is amiss.

A drug-seeking patient may complain of pain at level 10 on a 10 level rating scale. By all means document the complaint but add, if you observe it, that the patient was also cheerfully talking on the phone, going out for a smoke, etc.

Although it might not be considered behavior per se, muscle tone and movements should be noted – for example, myoclonic jerks may be caused by meperidine toxicity (Lauterbach 1999).

Emotion – mood and affect

Mood refers to enduring emotional state. Affect refers to the *observable* expression of feeling or emotion (Serby 2003). Affect may be fleeting, registered at the time by the patient's tone of voice, facial expression, motor activity, and speech. In a sense mood is to affect as climate is to weather. The summer climate (mood) in Cherokee, Iowa is hot and humid but the weather (affect) on this particular summer day is cool and cloudy. Mrs. Johnson is generally in good spirits (emotional climate) but today is nervous (emotional weather) about the results of her husband's test. A person may be suicidally depressed (mood) yet *appear* cheerful (affect).

You may ask a patient, "How are your spirits?" "How's your mood?" "How are you feeling?" These all assess mood. Of course, the patient may not wish to "complain". A patient may be "down", or "blue" or "not so good", phrases which may indicate depression, anxiety, anger, or guilt.

Since you don't really know what these phrases mean to the patient you might wish to ask an open-ended question, i.e., a question which doesn't lead to a specific kind of answer. "Could you tell me more about it?" is an open-ended question, as is, "Is there anything else?" Close-ended questions begin to narrow the range of inquiry and possible responses. For example, "Are you worried?" "What are you worried about?"

Illness is often depressing and many ill patients are depressed (Goodwin *et al.* 2003). The word depression in this context may simply mean an unpleasant mood, a feeling of dejection or listlessness, which will resolve in a few days or weeks when the situation improves and which needs no treatment per se, except for the skillful, empathic attention of nurse and doctor. If a depressed mood lasts for weeks, is relatively persistent during the day, and if the hospitalized patient has lost interest in people, feels guilty, cries frequently or has thoughts of suicide, depression may be more serious (Cavanaugh *et al.* 1983).

How do you assess the seriousness of a patient's depression? Part of this is intuition on your part, of course, but there may be signs that further questioning is necessary. The seriously depressed patient may keep the shades drawn, interacting minimally with you or with visitors. You will want to know how the patient is feeling and you can start with the questions above.

> A depressed elderly man with a history of alcoholism was hospitalized for the treatment of lung cancer. Throughout his hospitalization, he asked for help for pain and insomnia. One morning he was found in bed, the plastic garbage can liner over his head. He had taken his accumulated stash of opioids and sleeping pills and committed suicide. No one, including his family, had understood the depth of his anguish. Probably no one had asked.

Are you concerned that asking these questions will "put ideas" into your patient's head, increasing the risk of suicide? Everyone knows what suicide is, and it is unlikely that your questions will increase the risk in a particular patient. The greater worry is that by not assessing suicide risk, the danger in a particular patient will be overlooked.

> A stoic 60-year-old man with multiple myeloma, and multiple spinal compression fractures appears depressed. His nurse asks him about suicidal thoughts. He admits that when he's in a lot of pain, he wants to die, but that when the pain is controlled, he wants to live. He says he'd never commit suicide. He has no history of depression and no family history. His nurse arranges for better pain control. He does not need suicidal precautions.

Suffering due to pain, nausea, dyspnea, fatigue, or fear may become intolerable even for the most stable and resolute of us. Strange as it may sound, the thought that suicide may be available as an escape can provide some psychological relief, even hope. In this book we are not addressing the ethical arguments for or against suicide, assisted or otherwise. We are simply reminding you that suicidal thoughts do not in and of themselves demand an immediate response from you. Suicidal plans, however, do.

Suppose the patient says he's depressed and you're worried. You ask the patient to tell you about it. You ask the patient what else is on his mind, etc. Now let's say you are more worried.

Consider asking in order the following set of questions to assess the possibility of suicide:

- "Do you ever feel so bad that life doesn't seem worth living?"
- "Have you considered taking your own life?"
- "Have you thought about *how* you might do this?"
- "Do you have the *means* to do this?"
- "Have you thought about *where* you might do this?"
- "Have you thought about *when* you might do this?"

If a patient has more than vague, fleeting wishes of death – which many people have when they have severe pain, malaise, nausea, and the like – then you may wish to communicate your concerns to the physician in charge, especially if your patient is thinking about drinking a bottle of whiskey in his garage while the car is running. And you will wish to reassess the mood of the patients with vague, fleeting wishes of death.

Anxiety is another uncomfortable mood state. Do not assume that it is simply a direct reaction to hospitalization. It may be due again to delirium, medications, pain, nausea, dyspnea, a preexisting anxiety disorder, etc. However, the hospital is often a disquieting place and most seriously ill patients at some time or another do worry about death and dying, pain, becoming disabled, going bankrupt, becoming a burden to their families, etc. You can broach the subject of anxiety. "You seem worried. Am I right? Do you want to talk about it?"

The causes of anger must be assessed. We refer more to this emotion in Chapter 7. Rarely would you need to ask the following questions:

- "Have you ever felt so annoyed with someone that you thought about killing them?"
- "Are you feeling this way about someone right now?"
- "Who is this person?"
- "How might you kill them?" "When?" "Where?"

Of course, these are uncomfortable questions, but they can be asked gently.

Euphoria, though it may make a person a pleasure to talk to, can be a sign of a serious problem, either mania or a reaction to drugs such as steroids that can affect a person's judgment (Plihal *et al*. 1996). If euphoria is coupled with the inability to sleep, the patient needs further assessment. Opioid-induced euphoria is not a problem unless behavior is disturbed. Note that delirium is not associated with euphoria. Delirious patients are miserable.

Irritability means easily disturbed by mild stimuli. It needs assessment. For example, you fluff up a patient's pillow and he barks, "Not like that!"

Speech

Is the patient's speech loud, soft, or normal in volume? Is it fast, slow, or normal in rate? Is it fluid, halting, stuttered, or scanning in rhythm? Is it tangential, circumstantial? Logical or illogical? Is it coherent? Does the patient have trouble finding words?

Note especially if it is slurred because slurred speech is often associated with drug (opioids, benzodiazepine) or alcohol intoxication.

Thoughts

Under the heading of "thoughts", we should be reminded especially to think of the following: suicidal and homicidal thoughts, discussed above; and delusional thoughts, which we will discuss here.

Delusions are fixed, false beliefs (Cummings 1985). By "fixed", we mean that the false beliefs cannot be shaken by logical argument or by evidence. By "false", we mean not merely that they are untrue but also that the overwhelming majority of people in the person's social group would also hold them untrue.

Let us illustrate what we mean when we say a fixed, false belief. Consider the following, admittedly preposterous, situation.

Your patient, Mr. Tuddoe, insists that there are drug smugglers in the next room and they plan to kill him. You walk Mr. Tuddoe next door and introduce him to ninety-year-old Mrs. Macintosh who is in bed with pneumonia. He allows that she seems innocent enough but insists that the smugglers were in there a while ago. Furthermore, because they've left a listening device in the wall of his room he refuses to sleep there another night. By now, you're pretty fed up with all this nonsense, so you dash out to the nurse's station for the ten-pound sledge hammer stored there for just such occasions, return to Mr. Tuddoe's room, and pulverize the wall to prove to him there is no listening device in it.

Perspiring but pleased with yourself you motion with an upturned palm at the dust on the floor where the wall used to be and say, "See! I told you. No microphone."

"They got it out," he says.

Delusions in psychiatric conditions such as schizophrenia may be bizarre – the notion that one is being controlled by alien forces through radio waves or that one's thoughts are being broadcast, or that the television has special messages – or maybe more prosaic, such as the belief that people are plotting to do one harm (Nakaya *et al.* 2002).

In the delirious hospital patient, delusions may be bizarre or mundane. A patient may report that the nurses had a wedding party in the hall last night, that children and a cat were playing in the corner of the room, or, more ominously, that all the "nurses" who came into the room were impostors intent on doing the patient harm.

As we have illustrated, delusions cannot be shaken by evidence or argument. It is futile to explain that weddings aren't allowed in the hospital; that children, not to mention cats, may not spend the night in the room; that impostors would be identified as such.

Delirium, dementia, medications, delusional states due to medical disorders, and psychotic illnesses are all associated with hallucinations and delusions (Fricchione *et al.* 1995). We suggest you routinely screen for these with one simple question, a question we have found easy to ask because it is unobtrusive: "Did anything unusual happen last night?"

To screen for paranoia, the delusional belief of persecution, ask, "Has anybody been against you, been giving you a hard time, or accusing you of things?" "Are people too critical of you?"

If your patient has schizophrenia you may wish to ask, "Are you able to read people's thoughts?" "Are your thoughts being broadcast?" "Are you getting special messages from the TV?" "Are you being controlled by unseen forces?"

Perception

The most worrisome perceptual difficulties in the general hospital are hallucinations, perceptions of objects where none exist: smoke, water, birds, children, wedding cakes, boats, balloons, zombies, picnics, ants, fields and streams, cats, rubber duckies, Sherman tanks, and so forth. Visual hallucinations occur frequently in seriously ill patients, especially those with delirium (Cummings 1985; Fricchione *et al.* 1995; Webster and Holroyd 2000; Wancata *et al.* 2003). An illusion is related to a hallucination, except that an object is present but misperceived: folds in the sheets seen as insects; a mirror seen as a pool of water; or those ubiquitous, helium filled, silver gift balloons seen as a human heads.

> After her extubation, a 50-year-old woman with severe lung disease reported her "out of body experience". She said, "it was like I was walking along this road with my ex-husband, his wife and his mother. This sounds crazy but we turned into fish. We swam under a bridge and part of us were fish and I was aware I could breathe and the light was so bright, you wouldn't believe it. The water was like gold. It was sunrise or sunset under the bridge."

Auditory hallucinations – usually of voices – occur more frequently among patients with primary psychiatric disturbances (schizophrenia, manic-depressive illness, and major depression) than among hospitalized medical and surgical patients.

Tactile, kinesthetic, and olfactory hallucinations also occur among hospitalized medical patients and patients with psychiatric illnesses, but we will not discuss them here as visual hallucinations are generally much more frequent.

Delirium due to infection, surgery, drugs, etc., is the chief cause of hallucinations in the general hospital. Opioids may cause colorful, cartoon-like hallucinations.

If a person has a hallucination but doesn't believe the object was real, the person is not delusional. "I saw a cat in my room but I know that can't be true." Contrast this with "I heard the nurses having a wedding party last night. They should be ashamed." The second patient believes the nurses had a party in the hallway. He is delusional.

> A man in his 30's developed a post-operative delirium after pancreatectomy. He recalls being on ". . . the Oprah Winfrey show . . . in a place where they were using drugs. . . . They were filming." His delirium has now cleared and he knows he was experiencing hallucinations and delusions.

Recall this question for eliciting reports of such bizarre experiences: "Did anything unusual happen last night?" If the patient is unsure of what you mean or if you suspect delirium despite a denial of unusual events, you should ask, "Did you see or hear anything out of the ordinary?"

Reasoning

Reasoning may include abstract thinking, problem solving, visuospatial ability, judgment, insight, executive capacity, speed of processing, attention, and so on. We mention only a few things to look for.

- Does the patient understand instructions and follow them?
- How is the patient's judgment regarding day-to-day activities in the hospital?

Asking a patient to draw a clock can be used to screen for cognitive impairment, including executive function, speed of processing, and visuospatial reasoning (Juby et al. 2002). There are several ways to do this (Shulman 2000). Here, we describe the one we're most familiar with (Manos and Wu 1994; Manos 1997).

Using a round template, a compass, or a plastic sour cream cover, use a pen to trace a 4½ inch (11.4 cm) diameter circle on a piece of paper, preferably in the patient's chart. Explain: "When patients are in the hospital, they have trouble concentrating. I'd like to see how your concentration is. Would you please write the numbers in the face of a clock?" Wait until the patient has done so, and then say, "Would you make the clock say ten minutes after eleven?"

The clock is scored using the template or by dividing the clock into halves, using a straight edge to draw a line through the number 12 and the center of the circle, then into quarters, then into eighths. One point is given for the 1, 2, 4, 5, 7, 8, 10, and 11 in the proper octant of the circle relative to the number 12. One point is given for a little hand on the 11 and one for a big hand on the 11. No points for hands of approximately equal length.

Less than 8 points indicates cognitive impairment less than 5 points, prominent impairment.

The drawing of a deranged clock in the patient's chart is a graphic reminder of potential problems in patient management, patient education, and patient compliance.

A clear plastic disk, 4½ inches in diameter, marked into eighths, can easily be constructed and used repeatedly not only to draw the circle, but to score the clock as well. To do this, place one of the lines through the number 12 so that correctly placed numbers fall within the proper eighth of the circle (Figure 1).

Two other aspects of reasoning are insight and judgment (Feher *et al*. 1989; Fennig *et al*. 1996). Insight into psychotic disorders has generally meant that the patient is aware he has a mental illness, accepts the need for treatment, and understands that symptoms are due to his illness (Fennig *et al*. 1996). In the general hospital, a patient may or may not have insight into his delirium, hallucinations, depression, anger, or disruptiveness. Simple questions help assess insight:

- "Do you think you're having trouble remembering things?"
- "Do you think that party you heard in the hallway last night actually happened?"
- "What do you think caused you to have that experience?"
- "Do you feel safe here?"

A patient's judgment is assessed by observation and questioning. Does the patient continue to get out of bed without using the call light, despite several falls? Does the patient spit out pills rather than discussing why he won't take them?

Orientation

Be gentle and introduce the idea of testing:

- "When people are in the hospital, they can lose track of things. Let me ask you, do you remember the name of this place?"
- "And what city is that in?"
- "What would you guess the date is today?"
- "The day of the week?"

If the patient is disoriented to place, you may correct them like this: "Would you be surprised if I told you that you're in Virginia Mason Hospital in Seattle?"

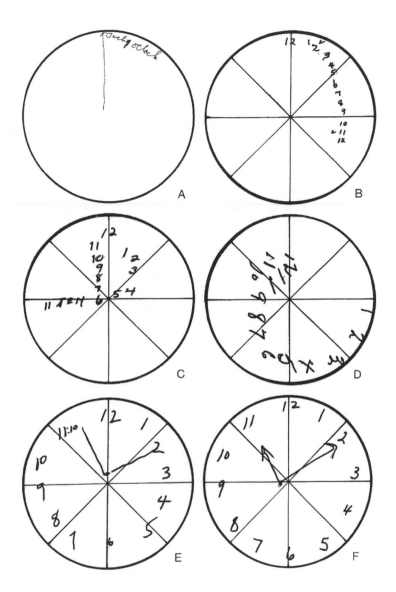

Figure 1 Scoring of the ten-point clock test on examples of clocks drawn by patients. (A) Score = 0 (B) The number 1 is in the correct octant; score = 1. (C) Numbers 1 and 11 are in the correct octants; score = 2. (D) Numbers 7, 8, 10, and 11 are in the correct octants; score = 4. (E) Numbers 1, 2, 4, 5, 7, 8, 10, and 11 are in the correct octants; score = 8. No points for hands of equal length. (F) Numbers 1, 2, 4, 5, 7, 8, 10, and 11 are in the correct positions. The little hand is on the 11 (1 point) and the big hand is on the 2 (1 point); score = 10 points.

Memory

You can assess memory by asking the patient what the doctors have explained to her about her problem. It is helpful to ask the patient to repeat the instruction or information you just provided.

> "Mrs. Hoosis, I'd like to know if I'm being clear. Could you repeat what I told you?"

Short-term memory testing is uncomfortable for the nurse as well as for the patient. It is a threat to the patient's sense of integrity, her sense of being sound or unimpaired. Although the examiner should always gently introduce testing, with memory testing in particular, care must be exercised.

> "Mrs. Hoosis, when people are ill they have trouble remembering things. I'd like to test your memory. I'm going to tell you the name of a friend of mine, his street address, and his favorite color and see if you can remember them. Don't worry. If you forget, I'll repeat them.
> "My friend's name is Roger Buskirk. What's my friend's name?"
> "Roger Buster."
> "Roger Buskirk."
> "Oh, Roger Buskirk."
> "Yes, and his address is 202 Pine Street. What's his street address?"
> "202 Pine Street."
> "Good. And his favorite color is blue. What's his favorite color?"
> "Blue."
> You have checked to make sure the patient has *registered* the information. You wait five minutes and then ask:
> "Do you remember the things I told you a little while ago?"
> "What things?"
> "What was my friend's name?"
> "Roger Pinecrest"
> "What was his street address?"
> "Pine Street."
> "What was his favorite color?"
> "Blue."

After you have administered this simple test to many patients, you will have developed a sense of what is normal and what is abnormal. You may wish to use your own friend's name, address, and favorite color. Some people offer the patient three words to remember and ask for them in five minutes.

There are a number of brief memory tests available (Pfeiffer 1975; Knopman and Ryberg 1989; Rankin 2000; Morrow and Ryan 2002) but as the patient's nurse for 8 to 12 hours a shift, you will have noticed the patient's problem with memory without formal testing and you should document it in your notes. Just writing "forgetful" is helpful to those using your notes but more specificity is better: "Forgets to use the call light." "Forgets that I've just been in." "Forgets she's taken her pills." "Forgets an IV is attached to her." "Forgets she has a Foley catheter." "Forgot her son was in to visit."

There are other approaches to the mental status examination, which include tests of memory, though nurses are often too busy to formally administer them (Folstein *et al.* 1975; Pfeiffer 1975; Kaufman and Zun 1995; Minarik 1995; Brackley 1997; Spreen 1998; Aird and McIntosh 2004; Gonzalez *et al.* 2004).

A few things to look for

The first order of business in dealing with difficult older patients may be to check that they are cognitively intact, i.e., that they do not have a dementia or a delirium. You will gently check orientation, ask about unusual nocturnal experiences, assess short-term memory, etc., and perhaps administer the ten-point clock test.

If you know that Mr. Sharp is normally oriented, alert, without nocturnal hallucinations, able to remember what you and the doctors tell him, able to draw a good clock, etc., you have that many more ways of assessing a change in mental status and need not ascribe his anger to dementia or delirium.

If the patient's memory and orientation are okay, but he is seeing frightening things at night and is paranoid, you need to know.

The patient may be intoxicated with slurred speech, poor memory, and ataxia.

You need to know.

You must be comfortable asking the questions to assess thoughts of suicide and with a little practice you will be.

You need not ask all patients all these questions (Table 2), but when you are worried about a troublesome patient, you should be able to assess the patient's mood and cognition to get a sense of why he's behaving the way he is. Document your findings in plain, concrete language. Examples and illustrations always help.

Table 2 Mental status assessment questions

For suicidal thoughts

- "Do you ever feel so bad that life doesn't seem worth living?"
- "Have you considered taking your own life?"
- "Have you thought about *how* you might do this?"
- "Do you have the *means* to do this?"
- "Have you thought about *where* you might do this?"
- "Have you thought about *when* you might do this?"

For hallucinations and delusions

- "Did anything unusual happen last night?"
- "Did you see or hear things that were frightening?"
- "Has anyone been giving you a hard time or been too critical of you?"

For orientation

- "When people are ill they have trouble remembering things. Do you recall the name of this place? What would you guess the date is? The day of the week?"

For memory

- "When people are ill they have trouble remembering things. I want to see how your memory is." Ask the patient to remember a name, an address, and a color. Repeat them until the patient remembers them. In three to five minutes ask the patient for the name, the address, the color.

continued

Table 2 (cont)

(alternatively, after you have explained something to the patient:)

- "When people are ill they have trouble remembering things. Could you repeat for me in your own words what I just told you?"

or

- "Could you repeat for me what the doctor told you about . . ." (your condition, the treatment plan, the operation, etc.)

Bibliography

Aird T. McIntosh M. 2004 Nursing tools and strategies to assess cognition and confusion. *British Journal of Nursing.* 13(10):621–6, May 27–Jun 9.

Brackley MH. 1997 Mental health assessment/mental status examination. *Nurse Practitioner Forum.* 8(3):105–13, Sep.

Buckley C. Curtin DM. Docherty J. Eustace P. 1987 Ageing and alpha 1 adrenoceptors in the iris. *Eye.* 1 (Pt 2):211–16.

Carter DM. Mackinnon A. Copolov DL. 1996 Patients' strategies for coping with auditory hallucinations. *Journal of Nervous & Mental Disease.* 184(3):159–64, Mar.

Cavanaugh S. Clark DC. Gibbons RD. 1983 Diagnosing depression in the hospitalized medically ill. *Psychosomatics* 24(9):809–15.

Cummings JL. 1985 Organic delusions: phenomenology, anatomical correlations, and review. *British Journal of Psychiatry.* 146:184–97, Feb.

Feher EP. Doody R. Pirozzolo FJ. Appel SH. 1989 Mental status assessment of insight and judgment. *Clinics in Geriatric Medicine.* 5(3):477–98, Aug.

Fennig S. Naisberg-Fennig S. Craig TJ. 1996 Assessment of insight in psychotic disorders. *Israel Journal of Psychiatry & Related Sciences.* 33(3):175–87.

Ferrando SJ. Eisendrath SJ. 1991 Adverse neuropsychiatric effects of dopamine antagonist medications. Misdiagnosis in the medical setting. *Psychosomatics.* 32(4):426–32, Fall.

Folstein MF. Folstein SE. McHugh PR. 1975 "Mini-mental state". A practical method for grading the cognitive state of patients for the clinician. *Journal of Psychiatric Research.* 12(3):189–98, Nov.

Fricchione GL. Carbone L. Bennett WI. 1995 Psychotic disorder caused by a general medical condition, with delusions. Secondary "organic" delusional syndromes. *Psychiatric Clinics of North America.* 18(2):363–78, Jun.

Gonzalez M. de Pablo J. Fuente E. Valdes M. Peri JM. Nomdeleu M. Matrai S. 2004 Instrument for detection of delirium in general hospitals: adaptation of the confusion assessment method. *Psychosomatics.* 45(5):426–431.

Goodwin RD. Kroenke K. Hoven CW. Spitzer RL. 2003 Major depression, physical illness, and suicidal ideation in primary care. *Psychosomatic Medicine.* 65(4):501–5, Jul–Aug.

Hennelly ML. Barbur JL. Edgar DF. Woodward EG. 1998 The effect of age on the light scattering characteristics of the eye. *Ophthalmic & Physiological Optics.* 18(2):197–203, Mar.

Jones C. Griffiths RD. Humphris G. Skirrow PM. 2001 Memory, delusions, and the development of acute posttraumatic stress disorder-related symptoms after intensive care. *Critical Care Medicine.* 29(3):573–80, Mar.

Juby A. Tench S. Baker V. 2002 The value of clock drawing in identifying executive cognitive dysfunction in people with a normal Mini-Mental State Examination score. *Canadian Medical Association Journal.* 167(8):859–64, Oct 15.

Kaufman DM. Zun L. 1995 A quantifiable, Brief Mental Status Examination for emergency patients. *Journal of Emergency Medicine.* 13(4):449–56, Jul–Aug.

Knopman DS. Ryberg S. 1989 A verbal memory test with high predictive accuracy for dementia of the Alzheimer type. *Archives of Neurology.* 46(2):141–5, Feb.

Lader M. 1983 The psychophysiology of anxiety. *Encephale.* 9(4 Suppl 2):205B–210B.

Lauterbach EC. 1999 Hiccup and apparent myoclonus after hydrocodone: review of the opiate-related hiccup and myoclonus literature. *Clinical Neuropharmacology.* 22(2):87–92, Mar–Apr.

Manos PJ. Wu R. 1994 The Ten Point Clock Test: A quick screen and grading method for cognitive impairment in medical and surgical patients. *International Journal of Psychiatry in Medicine.* 24(3) 229–44.

Manos PJ. 1997 The utility of the ten-point clock test as a screen for cognitive impairment in general hospital patients. *General Hospital Psychiatry.* 19(6):439–44, Nov.

Minarik PA. 1995 Cognitive assessment of the cardiovascular patient in the acute care setting. *Journal of Cardiovascular Nursing.* 9(4):36.

Moe PG. Seay AR. 2003 Neurologic and muscular disorders. In *Current Pediatric Diagnosis and Treatment.* Hay WW. Hayword AR. Levin MJ. Sondheimer JM, *et al.* Eds. New York: Lange Medical Books/McGraw-Hill.

Morency CR. 1990 Mental status change in the elderly: recognizing and treating delirium. *Journal of Professional Nursing.* 6(6):356–64.

Morrow LA. Ryan C. 2002 Normative data for a working memory test: the four word short-term memory test. *Clinical Neuropsychologist.* 16(3):373–80, Aug.

Nakaya M. Kusumoto K. Okada T. Ohmori K. 2002 Bizarre delusions and DSM-IV schizophrenia. *Psychiatry & Clinical Neurosciences.* 56(4):391–5, Aug.

Pfeiffer E. 1975 A short portable mental status questionnaire for the assessment of organic brain deficit in elderly patients. *Journal of the American Geriatrics Society.* 23(10):433–41, Oct.

Pickworth WB. Welch P. Henningfield JE. Cone EJ. 1989 Opiate-induced pupillary effects in humans. *Methods & Findings in Experimental & Clinical Pharmacology.* 11(12):759–63, Dec.

Plihal W. Krug R. Pietrowsky R. Fehm HL. Born J. 1996 Corticosteroid receptor mediated effects on mood in humans. *Psychoneuroendocrinology.* 21(6):515–23, Aug.

Rankin EJ. 2000 Bedside evaluation of learning and memory: descriptive information on a shortened version of the Luria Memory Words Test. *Journal of Clinical Psychology.* 56(1):113–18, Jan.

Serby M. 2003 Psychiatric resident conceptualizations of mood and affect within the mental status examination. *American Journal of Psychiatry.* 160(8):1527–9, Aug.

Shulman KI. 2000 Clock-drawing: is it the ideal cognitive screening test? *International Journal of Geriatric Psychiatry.* 15(6):548–61, Jun.

Spreen O. 1998 *A Compendium of Neuropsychological Tests.* Oxford: Oxford University Press.

Wancata J. Windhaber J. Krautgartner M. Alexandrowicz R. 2003 The consequences of non-cognitive symptoms of dementia in medical hospital departments. *International Journal of Psychiatry in Medicine.* 33(3):257–71.

Webster R. Holroyd S. 2000 Prevalence of psychotic symptoms in delirium. *Psychosomatics.* 41(6):519–22, Nov–Dec.

Chapter 2

Substance abuse

In this chapter we will provide you with information to make less daunting the care of patients who are abusing or are dependent on substances.[1] For the general hospital nurse these patients are challenging when behavior related to the substance creates an obstacle to the provision of good nursing care, our view, again, of what makes a patient "difficult". Sometimes patients demand drugs, or are dangerously intoxicated by them, or are withdrawing from them. We do not discuss the details of assessment and long-term treatment of chemical dependence though we include here a section on obtaining the proper care for these patients.

Substance *abuse* refers to a maladaptive pattern of drug use over a period of twelve months[2] causing significant distress or clinical impairment. The Diagnostic and Statistical Manual of Mental Disorders (DSM IV1994) provides the formal criteria. It will suffice for our purposes to list[3] some of the possible elements in the history of a person who might be suspected of having such a problem: substance-related absences from work or school; neglect of family responsibilities; driving a car while intoxicated; substance-related arrests for disorderly conduct; or continued use despite substance related recurrent discord with a partner or friend. One need not make a formal diagnosis to get a sense from the history that a patient may have a drug problem.

Substance *dependence* also refers to a maladaptive pattern of use over 12 months meeting the criteria of abuse but, as the name dependence implies, with the addition of loss of control over the use of the substance. Again we will not list the formal criteria because the nurse will be confronted with the practical problem of management far more frequently than with the need to make a formal diagnosis. Nevertheless, we again list some possible salient features from the history of a patient who might be suspected of being drug dependent: tolerance of quantities of the drug that would cause severe intoxication in a non-dependent person; a history of withdrawal[4] from the substance; visiting multiple doctors or driving long distances; continued use despite recognition of adverse health consequences.

The use of any illicit substance in the hospital can cause disruption in the patient's care but generally the narcotics and benzodiazepines cause the most trouble. This is simply because they are not only drugs of abuse but of therapeutic value as well and it is the nurse who administers them. Amphetamines, cocaine, and psilocybin mushrooms will not be ordered prn, around-the-clock, or any other way.[5]

In this chapter, then, our attention is focused on narcotics and benzodiazepines. We discuss alcohol elsewhere.

An ethical approach to patients often demands a patient-centered approach (Russell *et al.* 2003), but as we discuss elsewhere in this book, sometimes a conflict arises between the ethical principle of beneficence and the ethical principle of respect for patient autonomy (Woodward 1998). This conflict arises frequently in the care of the patients we are now about to discuss. The patient wants a drug, which if administered, will be harmful. If the patient's autonomy is respected, the nurse will not be acting with beneficence.

The patient who demands narcotics

Most experienced clinicians agree that undertreatment of pain remains a significant problem. The literature is robust (Resnik *et al.* 2001; Vallerand 2003). Nothing said in this chapter should be construed as suggesting that it is sometimes acceptable to deny a patient clinically appropriate and adequate opioid analgesia. The behavior of some patients, however, makes difficult the achievement of this humane goal.

The physiologic signs associated with acute pain are often absent in chronic pain syndromes, especially those caused by cancer (Carnevali and Reiner 1990). Nurses are taught that a patient's report of pain is often, if not always, the best measure of its presence and intensity (Broyles and Korniewicz 2002). Nurses, however, are sometimes confused when trying to apply this generally sound principle to the patient who exaggerates his pain or lies about it in an attempt to receive more narcotics or other intoxicants. If they conflict, should the nurse believe her clinical intuition or should she believe what the patient says?

> Because of the nursing shortage, Pam Green, R.N., who usually works on the oncology floor, has been temporarily assigned to the surgical floor. Eddie Edwards, forty, an unemployed shipyard worker admitted with a thigh abscess and cellulitis, calls Pam into his room.
>
> "This leg's killing me."
>
> "I'm sorry. I'll get you some more oxycodone. Be back in a minute."
>
> "No, not that, please. It makes me sick. I really need the morphine."
>
> "Eddie, Dr. Wang wants you to start taking your medicine by mouth. You can't go home on intravenous pain killers, you know."
>
> "Hey, I'm with you a hundred percent, but I can't take that stuff right now. I just threw up this morning."
>
> "Oh, you didn't tell me that."
>
> "It wasn't much."
>
> "You should tell me if you're throwing up."
>
> "Yeah, I will. Listen, I can't get up and walk with my leg hurting like this and Dr. Wang said I needed to get up so I wouldn't get a blood clot."
>
> "Alright, I'll get you some morphine."
>
> "I need ten. Five isn't enough."
>
> Returning to the room, Pam finds Mr. Edwards, dozing.
>
> "Eddie."
>
> "Uh, yeah . . ."
>
> "I have your morphine."
>
> "Ten?"

"Yes."

"Great."

An hour and a half later, not seeing Mr. Edwards up in the hall, Ms. Green returns to his room to find him nodding, the non-infected leg dangling over the edge of the bed, the newspaper comic section strewn over the floor. As she lifts the leg back onto the bed, he awakens.

"The leg's still killing me. I don't think the antibiotic is working. I need some more medicine."

"I think you ought to try the pain pills."

"I don't want to throw up."

She returns with the morphine to find that he's nodded off again so she approaches the bed.

"Eddie . . . Eddie." He arouses. "I brought you the morphine."

"Great."

After examining the patient's wound at the end of the shift, Dr. Wang comes by to talk to Nurse Green.

"The wound looks good. There's no erythema or swelling in the leg and he's afebrile. We'll send him home tomorrow. But he's pretty sedated. He shouldn't need that much morphine. Why don't you start tapering the doses?"

Dr. Wang doesn't change the orders.

At the change of shift, Ms. Green tells the evening nurse the plan but during the night Mr. Edwards complains bitterly about pain, receives more IV morphine, and falls while trying to go to the bathroom. He suffers a Colles' fracture, prolonging his hospital stay. Dr. Wang thinks Ms. Green is responsible for the fiasco.

Patients may demand narcotics for reasons other than the relief of pain (Peteet and Evans 1991). Drug dependent patients often deal with anxiety by taking drugs and since admission to a hospital makes most people anxious these patients seek drugs. The patient addicted[6] to narcotics may fear withdrawal and doubt the medical staff will protect him from it. A patient may wish oblivion through narcosis to escape the stress of hospitalization or seek the intense euphoria that intravenously administered opioids could provide.

Although the terms "addicted", "drug dependent", "substance dependent", etc., may evoke the image of an obnoxious person, the image is most often false. These are people like us but whose lives have been more painful than ours and whose emotional and social resources are scarce. Narcotics bring them surcease of suffering, albeit only briefly. In the general hospital, though, a minority of them cause disruptions, especially if they are dependent on intravenously administered narcotics. Their craving and fears, then, are all the more powerful. The drug dependent patient may angrily complain that he's in pain and nobody is listening or insist he's in narcotic withdrawal. He may threaten to leave the hospital. Rarely, he will threaten violence or suicide. His visitors may be loud and unruly. These extreme behaviors, as noted, are rare.

These patients become difficult when goals conflict: their chief goal of obtaining narcotics and your chief goal of providing good nursing care, in other words, when their behaviors present an obstacle to the provision of good nursing care.

If you focus excessively on preventing abuse of narcotics while the patient is under your care, you will be frustrated. It is best, instead, to focus on the medical problem and nursing needs rather than the drug problem per se. The most common problem of intravenous drug abusers is infection – cellulitis, endocarditis, hepatitis, AIDS, etc. A pattern of drug abuse in the hospital, then, is only a problem if it interferes with proper nursing and medical care of the problem that brought the patient to the hospital in the first place.

An intoxicated patient might dislodge IV's or pick at bandages; a somnolent patient has an increased risk of having a deep vein thrombosis, aspiration pneumonia, or a fall. The patient constantly pushing the call button is more than just a nuisance: this behavior may engender resentment in the nurse that may affect her clinical judgment. But if a patient is mildly sedated, but generally cooperative, moving about sufficiently in bed, with good balance, not choking on his food, etc., narcotic overuse in the hospital is not necessarily a problem or, at least, not a major problem, though it may impair the patient's judgment and impede discharge planning. With such patients, though, one must choose one's battles. These same docile patients might be irritable and angry were their sedation less.

You should not, of course, abandon attempts to reduce the amount of narcotics used – a goal for any patient since narcotics impair thinking, cause constipation, affect blood pressure, decrease respiratory drive, etc. It is especially important to switch from intravenous to oral opioids as soon as possible. The intravenous route is associated with shorter duration of action; steeper swings in blood concentration; increased risk of complications such as infection, bleeding, phlebitis; and increased burden on the nursing staff looking after intravenous paraphernalia.

Recall that most of these patients are in the hospital because of infection and that most of their pain is acute rather than chronic so that you may use objective methods to assess pain. Tachycardia may be caused by infection or pain, but a normal heart rate may help reassure you that pain is not excruciating. The same may be said for blood pressure. Look at the patient's pupils. Large pupils are caused by sympathetic discharge as may be caused by pain. Narcotics make the pupils small. So if a patient is fully alert, complaining of pain, and has large pupils, he may be insufficiently medicated. If pupils are small and the patient appears sleepy when observed without his knowledge, you may have some objective evidence for the efficacy of your analgesic approach.

Prn (as needed) vs. Around-the-clock (routine) Orders

If a patient who is addicted to narcotics has prn narcotic orders, it is likely he will have a complaint at the time the prn narcotic is due. What do you do, then, if the patient is asking for his prn morphine but you're worried that over-sedation threatens his well-being since he has been somnolent all day long, even tripping occasionally when out of bed and is described by the night shift as "forgetful"? If you deny the patient his morphine, he will be angry with you. If you administer it, you are putting him at risk.

This headache – your headache – can be remedied. Get the doctor to write around-the-clock narcotic orders and discontinue the prn orders. We repeat – get the doctor to write for routinely administered narcotics and discontinue the prn's. Routine orders take the struggle out of caring for the patient. Once the prn orders are discontinued, you gently, simply, calmly explain that the doctor has ordered the medication every four hours around the clock and that you will bring it even if the patient doesn't ask for it. You repeat when the next dose is due.

For this approach to work the following are necessary:

- First, a doctor willing to write the appropriate orders (i.e., around the clock not prn dosing), set limits with the patient, and assess the patient's response daily so adjustments can be made.
- Second, doses of narcotics sufficient to relieve pain, given frequently enough. Remember that the drug dependent patient will be tolerant to narcotics and will need higher doses – sometimes much higher – than other patients (Marie 1996).
- Third, a nurse willing to remain firm with the patient, and communicate to the next shift what the plan is.

Obviously, this plan will fail if the patient is suffering from significant, uncontrolled pain. The patient has come to us for help and we are, after all, in the business of providing relief of suffering as well as treatment of infection, etc. In determining which opioid to use, at which dose, etc., there is no substitute for clinical judgment. We can provide some guidelines, however:

- Help institute routinely scheduled, that is around-the-clock, opioid analgesia and discontinue prn analgesia.
- Work with the doctor and patient to switch from parenteral to oral medications as soon as possible. Consider rectal suppositories if the patient complains of vomiting.
- Prepare the patient for the change in regimens. "Tomorrow we're going to switch your medications from intravenous to oral. This will reduce the risk of infection, and inflammation of the veins."
- Consider using methadone both for analgesia and to prevent withdrawal (Mercadante *et al.* 2003).
- Avoid meperidine if possible because it is more likely to cause central nervous system toxicity (Latta *et al.* 2002).

The narcotics

A physician's experience will determine which narcotic analgesic is chosen. Table 3 lists the usually administered drugs along with some of their characteristics. For example, the duration of analgesia for *orally* administered morphine, codeine, oxycodone, meperidine, and hydromorphone is about four hours. A six-hour interval between oral doses is usually too long[7] to provide continuous analgesia. On the other hand, after methadone has been administered every four hours for two to three days, its duration of analgesia lengthens to six hours, making methadone a good choice for analgesia. A frequently held misconception is that methadone must be administered for days before it controls pain. Like the other narcotic analgesics, it works shortly after being taken.

Table 3 also indicates that the analgesic potency for all drugs is greater when given parenterally than orally. For example, 6 mg of oral morphine is generally considered

Table 3 Narcotic analgesics

	Equivalent analgesic parenteral/ oral dose	Duration[a] of analgesia of an oral dose (hours)	Parenteral dose equivalent to 10 mg of morphine	Duration[b] of analgesia in hours of IV or IM administration	
				IV	IM
Morphine sulfate	1/6[c]	4–5	10	2	4
Codeine sulfate	1/2 to 2/3	4–5	120	2	3–6
Hydromorphone	1/5	4–5	2	2	4–5
Meperidine	1/3 to 1/2	4–5	80–100	2	3–4
Oxycodone	1/2	4–5	10–15	2	4–5
Methadone	1/2	4 hours for the first three days, then 6 hours	10	2	4–5

Source: Gilman *et al.* 1985.

Notes
[a] Approximate duration
[b] Approximate duration
[c] In other words, 10 mg of parenteral morphine is roughly equivalent in analgesic potency to 60 mg of oral morphine in acute pain. All the equivalence numbers are approximate.

equivalent only to 1 mg of parenteral morphine for acute pain (Gilman *et al.* 1985). (The ration is 3 to 1 for chronic pain (Glare and Walsh 1991; Ashburn and Lipman 1993)). For methadone the oral to parenteral equivalence is 2 to 1. This makes several steps necessary in calculating a switch from an intravenous regimen of one drug to an oral regimen of a second drug. For example, 10 mg of IV morphine is equivalent to 10 mg of IV methadone, which is equivalent to 20 mg of oral methadone. Patients switched to methadone must be carefully monitored daily because of the danger of excessive build up of the drug.

Patient-controlled analgesia (PCA) in this group of patients may not have the desired effect of lowering total opioid used. The reason that PCA machines may diminish the amount of opioid used by the average, non-narcotic dependent patient is that when the patient controls his analgesia, fear of pain is diminished and hence the patient tolerates mild discomfort better. The narcotic dependent patient, on the other hand, is self-administering his opioid not only for pain relief but to achieve intoxication. It seems to generally be a bad idea to provide such patients with a high tech method for intravenous drug administration, but some patients will inevitably be provided with these machines, sometimes, perfectly appropriately as in certain patients with pancreatitis. The goal is to switch to oral medication as soon as possible.

Fentanyl patches (McEvoy 2003), providing a transdermal route, are used for chronic pain syndromes, especially those found in cancer patients. A *25-microgram* patch delivers 25 micrograms of fentanyl an hour but it is not all bioavailable, so even though it is 80 to 100 times more potent than morphine, such a patch over twenty-four hours is probably equivalent to 15 mg of IV morphine per 24 hours (90 mg of morphine orally in 24 hours). These patches are *inappropriate* for acute pain syndromes.

Physiologic dependence on and withdrawal from opioids

Let us turn for a moment to the question of physical dependence on opioids. Physical dependence implies that a narcotic withdrawal syndrome will develop when the drug is stopped, but withdrawal varies in intensity from mild to severe. People who have received large doses of opioids for long periods of time, such as heroin addicts, will have severe withdrawal reactions, whereas people who have received lower doses for shorter durations will have mild reactions or none at all.

What is a large dose of narcotic? What is a long period of time? What is a mild withdrawal syndrome? A severe withdrawal? We'll start with a description of narcotic withdrawal and then discuss the other questions.

Both the patient and the nurse may well overlook a mild withdrawal syndrome, as it will consist of a mild restlessness and insomnia that resolves without treatment in a few days. It is largely subjective. At the other end of the spectrum a narcotic addict in withdrawal (Slaby *et al.* 1978) will become anxious, crave the drug, and develop yawning, diaphoresis, lacrimation, and rhinorrhea – looking like someone with a bad case of the flu. Later there is pupillary dilatation, piloerection (i.e. goose flesh), muscle aches, decreased appetite, muscle twitches, and hot and cold flashes. In late withdrawal there may be autonomic hyperactivity (increased pulse, respiratory rate, and blood pressure), gastrointestinal disturbances (nausea, vomiting, diarrhea, weight loss), fever, and orgasm (Table 4).

Now, how much drug, by what route, for how long would it take to develop a physiologic dependence? Here is an approximate figure. If a 70 kilogram (154 lb) patient received 60 to 100 mg of parenteral morphine a day (or 600 to a 1000 mg of meperidine equivalents) for two weeks, she would develop a mild withdrawal syndrome on discontinuation of the drug – a syndrome that might be overlooked and which probably would need no treatment. Fear of addicting a patient should never interfere with adequate treatment of pain, especially since addiction and physiologic dependence are not the same thing. Addiction, also called substance dependence, requires a maladaptive pattern of use of the substance and a dominant focus on obtaining and using it. The cancer patient may be physiologically dependent on morphine but morphine use does not become the dominant focus of the patient's life.

Early identification and treatment of narcotic withdrawal can be crucial in forestalling agitation, anger, and acting out in opioid dependent patients. Nurses in large urban hospitals more frequently encounter this problem than their colleagues working elsewhere (Morrison *et al.* 2000). During entire careers many nurses may never see a case of *late* narcotic withdrawal. Intravenous drug users will be admitted to the hospital for a medical problem and they will receive narcotics for their pain and to prevent withdrawal. Many nurses may see very few, if any, cases of *early* withdrawal. They will, however, encounter narcotic dependent patients who tell them, either out of fear or in an attempt to receive larger or more frequent doses of narcotics, that they are in withdrawal. If the patient is able to sleep, rest quietly when unaware that she is being observed, and has normal or small sized pupils, is neither tachycardic, hypertensive, nor tachypneic the nurse can be fairly confident that serious withdrawal is not occurring. The chance that an addict could experience a significant withdrawal if treated with a total of 40 mg of oral methadone a day is very small (Gabbard *et al.* 2001).

Table 4 Narcotic withdrawal – symptoms and signs

Early opiate withdrawal

- Anxiety
- Drug craving
- Yawning
- Perspiration
- Lacrimation
- Rhinorrhea

Later

- Dilated pupils
- Piloerection (goose flesh)
- Myalgias
- Muscle twitches
- Decreased appetite
- Hot and cold flashes

Late withdrawal

- Fever
- Increased blood pressure
- Nausea and vomiting
- Weight loss
- Difficulty sleeping
- Orgasm
- Diarrhea
- Restlessness
- Increased pulse
- Increased respiratory rate and depth

Source: Slaby *et al.* 1978.

We revisit Nurse Green and Mr. Edwards after the patient's intravenous morphine has been discontinued.

"Pam, I'm in withdrawal. Look at my hands. They're shaking."

"I'm sorry you're feeling so poorly, Eddie, but I don't think you're in withdrawal. Your vital signs are stable and besides, you're receiving 60 mg of methadone a day which makes withdrawal almost impossible."

"I think I need more."

"Eddie, when you're sleeping your respiratory rate is 8 breaths a minute. I think the doctor will be reluctant to increase your dose for fear your respiratory drive will be depressed. You've got to keep breathing, you know. It's important for your health."

"Yeah. Yeah. All right."

Since pain, nevertheless may very well be a real issue, the methadone should be given in divided doses so that its duration of analgesia is taken advantage of, say 10 mg P. O. q 6 hours around the clock. A once-a-day dose is sufficient to prevent withdrawal but will not treat pain for 24 hours.

Patients may require larger or more frequent doses depending on circumstances, but for an abscess in the deltoid, for example, and a heroin habit, doses adequate for analgesia might range from as little as 5 mg P. O. q 4 hours to 30 mg P. O. q 4 hours. Ten mg of methadone P. O. q 4 hours is sufficient for most of the patients we have seen who are in the hospital for cellulitis. The interval *should* be increased to q 6 hours after two to three days. Of course, after surgical debridement requirements will increase and for patients who are dependent on large doses of narcotics who have undergone major surgery, such as pancreaticoduodenectomy (Whipple procedure), considerably higher doses of methadone may be necessary.

> Miss Moonbracelets, a 24-year-old homeless jewelry maker, was admitted to the hospital with a markedly erythematous and swollen right arm where she had been injecting heroin.
>
> She was placed on 10 mg of methadone every six hours around the clock with prn ibuprofen for pain. IV antibiotics were instituted.
>
> Over the weekend, she told the resident physician that she was going to leave the hospital unless her methadone dose was increased because she was in narcotic withdrawal. The dose was increased to 15 mg orally every 6 hours around the clock. Her fever had diminished but not fully resolved, the erythema had disappeared, and the swelling began to decline, but the patient again threatened to leave the hospital. Because of ongoing fever, a transesophageal echocardiogram had been planned to rule out endocarditis.
>
> Her pupils were small and she had been sleeping much of the day. An evening nurse described the patient as forgetful.
>
> This time the patient was told that the methadone would not be increased. The risks of leaving the hospital were explained. It was explained that if she left AMA she would be given no methadone for a self-tapering of narcotics at home. She agreed to stay and was discharged several days later.

Some patients attempt to reduce the stresses of hospitalization – the fear of procedures and of the unknown, of strangers, of social isolation, of unfamiliar routines and environs – by inappropriately sedating themselves.

> Ms. Debbie Crisp, a 23-year-old grocery clerk, had been repeatedly hospitalized for complications of Crohn's disease since childhood. As an outpatient, she used opioids infrequently, but during each hospitalization to obtain oblivion, she demanded high doses of intravenous hydromorphone, lorazepam, and diphenhydramine. Ms. Crisp growled and snapped at anyone suggesting a decrease in any of these medications, yet her over-sedation put her at risk for complications. Finally, firm but gentle limit setting was instituted – a concerted effort by her nurse, physician, house staff, and psychiatric consultant – allowing first a switch to oral medication, then a switch to routinely administered medication, then a step by step reduction in dose. Following this intervention, her hospital stays were shortened, in part, because she was no longer over-sedated, hence she was out of bed more, aiding her recovery and reducing the incidence of complications.

Of those making the effort to get the situation under control, the nurse is listed first. She was, in fact, the driving force in establishing a plan of action. She remained calm, friendly, and matter of fact when faced with the patient's anger, saying if verbally attacked, "I can see you don't feel so well right now. I'll come back in a while when you're feeling better."

Because Ms. Crisp's drug seeking was brought under control, and because the nurse could separate herself from the patient's abusive behavior, she did not dread taking care of her. With good humor, she insisted on examining the patient each day, even when the patient initially refused, coming back later to do it. One morning Ms. Crisp again complained of pain, and the nurse, quite familiar with the look and feel of the patient's abdomen, immediately recognized a new lump within it. Though Ms. Crisp's complaint seemed much like the others, the nurse knew something had changed. No delay was made in the diagnosis of a new small bowel obstruction.

Benzodiazepines and other sedative hypnotics

Benzodiazepines (Table 5) are a class of drugs that can reduce anxiety without causing sedation (Carrasco and Van de Kar 2003). They cause euphoria in some patients and they are potentially addicting. They are best used for short-term treatment of anxiety.

Although they may sometimes be used to relieve the anxiety associated with hospitalization, they should be avoided in most patients over the age of 65 because they impair balance and memory, and frequently cause confusion (Petrovic et al. 2003). These drugs are often associated with delirium in the elderly (Karlsson 1999).

In a cognitively intact patient whose anxiety is intolerable or who cannot sleep because of anxiety they can be helpful, but in cognitively impaired patients or those seeking surcease of sorrow through sedation, they are dangerous. Just as some patients

Table 5 Benzodiazepine comparison

	Equivalent oral dose (mg)	Daily oral range (mg)	Half-life (hours) Parent	Active metabolite
Long acting				
• Diazepam	5	6–40	20–50	yes[a], 50–100
• Chlordiazepoxide	10	15–100	5–30	yes, 50–100
• Chlorazepate	6.5–7.5	15–60	[b]	yes, 50–100
• Clonazepam[c]	0.5	1–3		yes
• Prazepam	10	20–60	78	yes, 50–100
• Flurazepam	30	15–60	[d]	yes, 50–100
Short acting				
• Oxazepam	15	30–120	5–10	no
• Lorazepam	1	2–6	10–20	no
• Alprazolam	0.5	0.75–4	12–15	yes, 12–15
• Temazepam	30	15–30	9–12	no
• Triazolam	0.5	0.25–10	2.2–4.5	yes, 3.9

Source: Lacy et al. 2003.

Notes
[a] Major metabolite is desmethyldiazepam.
[b] Hydrolyzed to desmethyldiazepam before absorption.
[c] Clonazepam may be thought of as a benzodiazepine though its structure is different.
[d] Rapidly metabolized to desalkyflurazepam.

may demand inappropriately high doses of narcotics to escape some may demand inappropriately high doses of benzodiazepines. Limit setting, oral administration, and regularly scheduled dosing as contrasted with prn dosing should be the plan.

Intravenous diphenhydramine can cause sedation and euphoria. It is sometimes a drug of abuse in the general hospital (Dinndorf *et al.* 1998).

Drug dependent patients can be trying, especially when they are surreptitiously taking drugs. You may need to search the patient's room for drugs.

> Mr. Glassy, a merchant marine seaman, admitted with falling episodes, is somnolent and inappropriate and you find an unidentified yellow capsule in his bed about which he claims ignorance. Dr. Avatar acknowledges the problem and asks for your help. You enter Mr. Glassy's room.
>
> "Mr. Glassy, sometimes when people are ill, they lose track of things and bring medications into the hospital that they forget about. I'd like to look through your things with you to see what medications you might have here."
>
> "You're not going to search my things, are you?"
>
> "We're going to look at them together."
>
> "How come?"
>
> "Because people sometimes forget what medicines they've brought in with them, and it's important for us to know. It's part of their medical history."
>
> "Oh."
>
> "Let's start here with your steamer trunk."
>
> A little while later, holding a bottle of yellow capsules, "What are these?"
>
> "Oh, I forgot about those. They're my relaxers."
>
> "We're going to put them in a safe place for you."

You asked *permission* to look through the patient's belongings *in his presence* (Plumeri 1984). Had the patient refused to let you go through his things in his presence, it would have been a red flag. We advise against surreptitious room searches. At discharge, Mr. Glassy's yellow relaxers will have to be returned to him, but it behoves you to know what they are and to warn the patient about them if appropriate. You should ask Dr. Avatar to confront the patient about drug abuse and see if professional help is available.

When you suspect that a patient is being supplied drugs by friends, it may be necessary to confront the patient with your suspicion, difficult as this often is. One uses a gentle tone but direct wording. "You know, the stress of hospitalization sometimes leads people to take drugs to relieve that stress, but we really can't allow it because it's too dangerous. People can stop breathing or have an accident if using drugs. We may be wrong about you, but we can't take the risk, so we'd like your visitors to check at the nursing station before going in to see you. We'd like you to leave the door open when you have visitors." It may be necessary to bar visitors entirely (Peteet and Evans 1991).

Mr. Glassy's yellow capsule may have been a barbiturate. Before the development of the much safer benzodiazepines, barbiturates were used as tranquilizers and sleeping pills, hence the category name sedative/hypnotics for an array of chemically dissimilar drugs.

Their relative sedating power is listed in Table 6. Taken at sufficient doses for long enough all may lead to a withdrawal syndrome if discontinued.

Table 6 Sedative hypnotic equivalents[a]

Drug	Oral dose (mg)
Diazepam	10
Whiskey (100 proof)	90 ml (3 oz.)
Secobarbital	100
Pentobarbital	100
Phenobarbital	30
Butalbital	50
Methaqualone	300
Glutethimide	500
Ethchlorvynol	750
Chloral hydrate	1000
Meprobamate	400

Source: Ready *et al.* 1980

Note
[a] Taken from the Virginia Mason Hospital pain cocktail prescription form.

Physiologic dependence on tranquilizers by definition means that a dependent person will develop a withdrawal syndrome when he stops taking the tranquilizers. This may be mild, with only anxiety and fragmented sleep, or severe with hypertension, tachycardia, fever, hallucinations and delusions, and seizures. Such a severe withdrawal reaction is similar to delirium tremens (see Chapter 3). The product of dose and duration of use of the tranquilizer determine the severity of withdrawal. So, for example, 30 mg of diazepam a day for a month might lead to a mild withdrawal or none at all if discontinued, but 50 mg for 6 months might lead to a more significant withdrawal. Of interest is the potency of some of the relatively new tranquilizers, like alprazolam, which is ten times more potent than diazepam. Alprazolam at 2 mg a day is like 20 mg of diazepam a day.

Note also that the shorter acting drugs often lead to a more severe withdrawal when discontinued because they are rapidly metabolized, allowing the brain little time to adapt, whereas the longer acting drugs leave the brain slowly, so adaptation has more time to occur.

Sometimes intensive care unit patients are treated with lorazepam, as much as 5–10 mg per hour for weeks. This is often an inappropriate treatment for the agitation of delirium, but it happens. These infusions can simply be turned off without fear of withdrawal. Apparently, enough lorazepam accumulates in tissues so that withdrawal is usually not a problem.

With limit setting, routinely scheduled drugs, an oral route, knowing what to look for, and a supportive managing physician, you need not dread substance dependent patients (Table 7).

Table 7 Intervention for excessive or illicit analgesic or tranquilizer use

Interventions	Examples
• Document your suspicions of illicit drug use	• Mr. Hatter appears intoxicated after his friends visit • Needles found in the room
• Document clinical observations of overmedication or other problems	• Mr. Willow sleeps most of the day • Ms. Nott appears comfortable when unaware she's being observed • Mr. Watt forgets what he's told • Ms. Blue yells at staff to bring her medication • Mr. Feld is unsteady on his feet
• The wording of explanations is important	• "We're going to bring your medication every four hours around the clock" • "Injections increase the risk of damaged veins, infection, and bleeding so we're going to switch to oral medication"
• If appropriate, discuss concerns about illicit drug use with the patient	• "You know, Mr. Hatter, we're concerned that you may be taking drugs that haven't been prescribed for you" • ". . . that your friends are bringing in drugs" • ". . . that you appear to be intoxicated" • "We really can't permit you to take illicit drugs in the hospital"
• You may need to search the patient's room in his presence	• "Sometimes people forget which medications they've brought in to the hospital with them. I'd like to go through your things with you to see what medications you may have brought in"

• If appropriate, keep the door open when friends visit

• You may need to have all visitors check in at the nurses' station to warn them against providing illicit drugs to the patient

• You may need to restrict patient to his room if illicit drug use endangers his health

Ask the physician to:

• discontinue prn medication

• have *necessary* medications given on a routine, i.e., scheduled basis

• switch from the IV or IM route to the to the P. O. or P. R. route

• consider oral methadone for analgesia

• speak with the patient about the change. Be present when the physician does so

An administrative approach

The appendix to the article by Peteet and Evans (1991) is a statement on their hospital's drug and alcohol-free environment, which is given to all patients. Following a preamble, which describes the hospital's wish to serve the patient's medical needs, six rules are stated:

- Staff may request permission to search your personal effects. You may choose to leave rather than consent to the search.
- Clinical staff may perform tests to determine if you are using drugs or alcohol. You may choose to leave rather than consent to such tests.
- If you are using substances, your physician will discuss options with you. If you continue to do so you may be discharged.
- Staff will prohibit or supervise your visitors if there are grounds to believe you are receiving illicit substances from them. Disruptive visitors will be asked to leave.
- Staff may confine you to your room or nursing unit to avoid substance abuse. If you leave the hospital without permission you may not be readmitted.
- The hospital will discharge you if you do not control behavior that endangers medical treatment or is physically assaultive or verbally threatening to staff, other patients, or visitors. You will be given a list of other hospitals in the area where you may obtain medical care.

These rules are a concrete illustration of limit setting. If a hospital's administration incorporates them, the nurse's job becomes easier. However, nowadays patients are often too ill to be discharged.

Concomitantly, hospitals whose patients often have substance abuse problems should have mechanisms for referring patients for treatment.

A nurse's experience over the years

A nurse we interviewed had this to say about drug seeking patients:

> "At the beginning of my career, I, like my colleagues, dreaded caring for narcotic seeking patients. To avoid conflict, we often allowed them to dictate their own care until things got completely out of control. Some patients demanding meperidine every half hour developed convulsions. Nurses might call physicians every half hour to come up and readdress a patient's pain complaint. I eventually learned to take charge early rather than waiting for a crisis. Conferences helped, as did consultants who knew about medications and aberrant behavior. I no longer mind caring for these patients because I know what to do. Initially they seek drugs but I respond differently than I used to and eventually they do too.
>
> "I assess the total clinical picture – medical, emotional, psychosocial – then develop a plan tailored to the individual patient. I was long unaware of this approach with narcotic seeking patients. Methods of caring for them do not appear widely disseminated and the medical community has a very hard time setting limits.
>
> "For example, I learned that Eddie D., the young man just assigned to me, had had a problem with drug dependence in the past. At eight in the morning I went

in with Dr. Lake to find the patient drooling and so sleepy that Dr. Lake was unable to shake him awake. 'Something's got to give,' he said, 'I'll stop the promethazine. He can have trimethobenzamide suppositories if he's nauseated.' I said that was fine.

"Then Dr. Lake walked away. And now comes a key issue, a critical thing I've learned. I looked at the written orders and he hadn't discontinued the promethazine. So I called after him, 'Dr. Lake, you didn't discontinue the promethazine.' And he said, 'Well, yes, I'll leave it there but just don't give it to him.'

"Telling the nurse not to give a medication but leaving it on order puts the nurse in the middle. If she does not administer the medication that is on order, the patient is angry with her. If she does, the doctor is angry with her. I don't allow myself to be in this fix anymore. I'll plead my case but as long as that promethazine is on order the patient will ask for it and I will give it. I'm not going to argue about it. If the doctor doesn't want it given, an order must be written to have it discontinued. My part of the bargain is to deal with the patient without constantly calling the doctor for requests for medication changes. Dr. Lake discontinued the promethazine order.

"The assessment part of nursing skills is so important in caring for drug seeking patients. Eddie D. is now sitting in his chair, talking, laughing, joking with someone on the phone, and says, as I come in, 'Oh, hang on a minute. Oh, by the way I want my promethazine for nausea. And bring in some ice chips,' then goes back to the phone and starts talking. Now this is unexpected behavior from a person who says he is as nauseated as Eddie claims. I remained for a while and he talked and he joked and was fine on the phone.

"I said, 'You know what, the promethazine has been discontinued, but I'll bring you a trimethobenzamide suppository.'

"And I did and he said, 'Get the hell out of here. . . .'

"A little later with encouragement, he was able to get up and shower and walked about. He did fine.

"When caring for these patients, your assessments need to be twice as thorough because their perception of things is so distorted that you can't rely on what you're told. So you'd better assess in the morning and check several times during the day.

"For example, Debbie Crisp was a 22-year-old woman with Crohn's who demanded and often received huge daily intravenous doses of hydromorphone, lorazepam, and diphenhydramine for weeks at a time as an escape. The day came, as it always does, when we changed her to oral medication. She wanted her IV medication, but I was comfortable telling her no. She did fine.

"In the morning, I examined her abdomen. It was soft. By noon, however, it was distended like a sausage, particularly on the right side, at the location of her anastamosis at the ileocecal valve. She reported more pain and nausea. I knew that she wasn't just drug seeking. I called Dr. K. He was great and came right over, arranging to dilate a stricture. She went home the next day.

"You have to follow someone like Debbie very closely because she always complains of pain and nausea. Thank heaven I looked at her in the morning and then at noon when her abdomen was dramatically different.

"Sometimes family members are more difficult than patients. Mr. Cramer, 49, in with pancreatitis, a drinker who'd been abstinent a few years by his report, had been here for five weeks. He demanded diazepam and a morphine PCA. He was able to get up and about when he wanted but he never got out of bed. Every day the doctors would write 'Ambulate T. I. D.' and he and I would have this go around, 'Bob, time to go for a walk.' No way. He wouldn't do it so finally one day, as he lay in bed coloring and painting, I simply asked. 'Why don't you ever get out of bed?' 'Because I've never had a month to just lie around before and I'm taking full advantage of it,' he said.

"He continued asking that his morphine PCA dose be upped, but then one day the doctors asked me to decrease it from one milligram an hour to half a milligram an hour. He'd be going home soon.

"At eight in the morning, his girlfriend, identifying herself as his wife called me, crying. 'You have to get in there. You're decreasing his medication and he's going through withdrawal and he's lying in that bed going crazy and he's crying right now and you guys gave him all these drugs and now you're going to let him go through withdrawal. You can't do this. You have to. . . .'

"I had spent a lot of time with him and I'd heard their phone conversations and knew she had a drinking problem.

"'You know Mrs. Cramer, I'll go in and take care of it right now.'

"Mr. Cramer was lying calmly in bed, but I thought maybe he really is scared of withdrawal. He's a bit of a character but still. Relying on what I'd learned about assessment for withdrawal, I checked his vital signs, his skin, his pupils – nothing was out of line. His vital signs were fine. He was calm. He wasn't diaphoretic.

"I talked to him. 'You know you're not going through withdrawal. We won't let you go through withdrawal. You're still getting your pain medicine. Every eight minutes, you can push that button. Your lorazepam is still ordered every four hours. I'll bring it to you every four hours. I'll keep a close eye on you today. I won't let you go through withdrawal.'

"After that he was fine. He didn't bother me any more about it, nor did Mrs. Cramer. Being aware of the proper assessment for narcotic withdrawal has given me confidence in situations such as these and in instilling confidence in my patients as well."

Concluding remarks

The preceding interview illustrates many of the ideas we have presented here. The nurse makes it her or his duty to learn about the potential for a particular patient to have a substance use disorder while in hospital – taking a history, getting the patient's view of the hospitalization. The patient's view of their condition and something of their living situation should be included in the history. Then the patient is examined with heightened attention because the nurse may later be unable to rely on the patient's reports. In addition to the usual parts of the physical evaluation, level of alertness, quality of speech, and pupillary size are noted.

Some mild intoxication or euphoria caused by the prescribed medications may not endanger the patient's health and safety in which case the nurse may decide to continue the current regimen without change. She will, of course, continue to monitor the patient's alertness, behavior, sleep, etc. The patient must be regularly examined.

The nurse who identifies potentially dangerous intoxication will naturally speak with the physician about it and help make a plan. Around-the-clock regimens are usually better than prn regimens. Methadone is often helpful because, after two or three days, the duration of analgesia is 6 hours. IV medications should be eliminated as soon as possible.

Nurses working in large city hospitals will also watch for the possibility of withdrawal, especially in patients with a known habit of intravenous drug use.

Patients and their families need education about drugs and the nurse will be the principal person to provide it. If the nurse has a sense of mastery in caring for these patients, their care can be as gratifying as the care of any other patient – sometimes more so because a human being has been helped despite the challenge.

Bibliography

Ashburn MA. Lipman AG. 1993 Management of pain in the cancer patient. *Anesthesia & Analgesia*. 76(2):402–16, Feb.

Bailes B. 1998 What perioperative nurses need to know about substance abuse. *AORN Journal*. 68(4):611–14, 617–22, 625–6, Oct.

Broyles LM. Korniewicz DM. 2002 The opiate-dependent patient with endocarditis: addressing pain and substance abuse withdrawal. *AACN Clinical Issues*. 13(3):431–51, Aug.

Carnevali DL. Reiner AC. 1990 *The Cancer Experience. Nursing Diagnosis and Management*, p. 399. Philadelphia: J. P. Lippincott Company.

Carrasco GA. Van de Kar LD. 2003 Neuroendocrine pharmacology of stress. *European Journal of Pharmacology*. 463(1–3):235–72, Feb 28.

Davis AJ. 1978 Brompton's cocktail: making good-byes possible. *American Journal of Nursing*. 78(4):610–12, Apr.

Dinndorf PA. McCabe MA. Friedrich S. 1998 Risk of abuse of diphenhydramine in children and adolescents with chronic illnesses. *Journal of Pediatrics*. 133(2):293–5, Aug.

Gabbard GO, *et al*. 2001 *Treatment of Psychiatric Disorders. American Psychiatric Press*. [on line] database title: STAT!Ref Online Electronic Medical Library, last accessed 7 Dec 2003 at http://online.statref.com/document.aspx?fxid=7&docid=145. Location in book: section 4, Methadone maintenance.

Gammaitoni AR. Fine P. Alvarez N. McPherson ML. Bergmark S. 2003 Clinical application of opioid equianalgesic data. *Clinical Journal of Pain*. 19(5):286–97, Sep–Oct.

Gilman AG. Goodman LS. Rall TW. Murad F. 1985 *Goodman and Gilman's The Pharmacologic Basis of Therapeutics*. 7th Edn. New York: Macmillan Publishing Company.

Glare PA. Walsh TD. 1991 Clinical pharmacokinetics of morphine. *Therapeutic Drug Monitoring*. 13(1):1–23, Jan.

Inturrisi CE. 2002 Clinical pharmacology of opioids for pain. *Clinical Journal of Pain*. 18(4 Suppl):S3–13, Jul–Aug.

Karlsson I. 1999 Drugs that induce delirium. *Dementia & Geriatric Cognitive Disorders*. 10(5):412–15, Sep–Oct.

Lacy CF. Armstrong LL. Goldman MP. Lance LL. 2003 *Drug Information Handbook*. 10th Edn. Cleveland, Ohio: Lexi Comp Inc. Am. Pharm. Assoc.

Latta KS. Ginsberg B. Barkin RL. 2002 Meperidine: a critical review. *American Journal of Therapeutics*. 9(1):53–68, Jan–Feb.

Marie B. 1996 Chemical abuse and pain management. *Journal of IV Nursing*. 19(5): 247–50.

McEvoy GK (ed.) 2003 *AHFS Drug Information. American Society of Health-System Pharmacists, Inc.* [on line] database title: STAT!Ref Online Electronic Medical Library, last accessed 7 Dec 2003 at http://online.statref.com/document.aspx?fxid=1$docid=772. Location in book: 28:00 Central nervous system agents, 28:08.08 opiate agonists, fentanyl citrate.

Mercadante S. Bianchi M. Villari P. Ferrera P. Casuccio A. Fulfaro F. Gebbia V. 2003 Opioid plasma concentration during switching from morphine to methadone: preliminary data. *Supportive Care in Cancer.* 11(5):326–31, May.

Morrison EF. Ramsey A. Synder BA. 2000 Managing the care of complex, difficult patients in the medical-surgical setting. *MEDSURG Nursing* 9(1):21–6.

Peteet JR. Evans KR. 1991 Problematic behavior of drug-dependent patients in the general hospital. A clinical and administrative approach to management. *General Hospital Psychiatry* 13:150–5.

Petrovic M. Mariman A. Warie H. Afschrift M. Pevernagie D. 2003 Is there a rationale for prescription of benzodiazepines in the elderly? Review of the literature. *Acta Clinica Belgica.* 58(1):27–36, Jan–Feb.

Plumeri PA (1984) The room search. *Journal of Clinical Gastroenterology* 6:181–5.

Ready B, *et al.* 1980 The management of chronic pain. *University of Davis Medicine.* 7 (13):13–24.

Resnik DB. Rehm M. Minard RB. 2001 The undertreatment of pain: scientific, clinical, cultural, and philosophical factors. *Medicine, Health Care & Philosophy.* 4(3):277–88.

Russell S. Daly J. Hughes E. Hoog Co. C. 2003 Nurses and 'difficult' patients: negotiating non-compliance. *Journal of Advanced Nursing* 43(3):281–7, Aug.

Schweizer E. Rickels K. 1998 Benzodiazepine dependence and withdrawal: a review of the syndrome and its clinical management. *Acta Psychiatrica Scandinavica, Supplementum.* 393:95–101.

Shir Y. Rosen G. Zeldin A. Davidson EM. 2001 Methadone is safe for treating hospitalized patients with severe pain. *Canadian Journal of Anaesthesia.* 48(11):1109–13, Dec.

Slaby AE. Lieb J. Tancredi LR. 1978 *Handbook of Psychiatric Emergencies.* Garden City, NY: Medical Examination Publishing Co., Inc.

Tucker C. 1990 Acute pain and substance abuse in surgical patients. *Journal of Neuroscience Nursing.* 22(6):339–49, Dec.

Vallerand AH. 2003 The use of long-acting opioids in chronic pain management. *Nursing Clinics of North America.* 38(3):435–45.

Wesson DR. Ling W. 2003 The Clinical Opiate Withdrawal Scale (COWS). *Journal of Psychoactive Drugs.* 35(2):253–9, Apr–Jun.

Woodward VM. 1998 Caring, patient autonomy and the stigma of paternalism. *Journal of Advanced Nursing.* 28(5):1046–52, Nov.

Chapter 3

Delirium

Edna McGunty, 75, suffering from arthritis and congestive heart failure, was admitted to the hospital this morning with pneumonia. She's been restless most of the day.

Don Dolbach, R.N., has just come on duty on the night shift and at 12:15 am goes in to check on her. Sitting at the edge of the bed, her gown up to her hips, she is entangled in the IV line, and trying to stand up.

"Just a minute, Mrs. McGunty, I'll help you with that."

Eyes fixed on her IV line, he does not notice her bare her teeth at him as he approaches, but when he touches her arm, she simultaneously spits at him and kicks him in the shins.

"Ow! Mrs. McGunty, what are you doing . . ."

"Oh, God! Oh, God! Don't let them! Don't. . . ."

"Mrs. McGunty, I'm your nurse . . ."

This time she scratches his arm. He moves back. She stands suddenly, knocking over the IV pole. Keeping an eye on her, he backs towards the door and calls down the hall.

"Hey, I need some help in here."

Eventually with the help of another nurse and a nurse's aid, he holds the patient still enough to administer first 1, then a little later, 2 mg of IV lorazepam. The patient falls asleep. They put a Posey vest on her.

She's awake and screaming an hour later. Lorazepam is administered intermittently through the night. In the morning Mrs. McGunty is difficult to arouse but when she finally wakes up, she's more confused but lethargic. The next night, however, the whole scenario repeats itself. Finally, IV haloperidol is substituted for lorazepam and the patient's agitation is controlled with much less sedation.

Agitated delirium

The confused, agitated patient is one of the most difficult to care for. Slapping, biting, pushing, punching, screaming, or simply refusing to allow anyone near her for fear of a plot against her, this patient is immune to rational argument, reassurance, and direction. This patient is dangerous to herself and to others.

The syndrome of disturbed consciousness and cognition developing over a period of hours to days is called delirium (American Psychiatric Association 1994). It has many synonyms including: encephalopathy, acute confusional state, acute brain syndrome, acute brain failure, acute organic psychosis, acute organic reaction, cerebral insufficiency, ICU psychosis, dysergastic reaction, organic brain syndrome, reversible cerebral dysfunction, reversible dementia, and others.

Delirium is a syndrome of disordered thinking and perception that is due to a medical problem, develops over hours to days, and usually resolves within days to weeks. The prevalence of delirium in some hospitals may be as high as 20%. It is especially high in older patients and patients with a dementia (Kolbeinsson and Jonsson 1993; Rockwood 1993; Fick *et al.* 2002; van der Mast 2003). Many of the delirious patients in a hospital become delirious shortly before admission (Manos and Wu 1997). All experienced general hospital nurses have seen the syndrome, but not all have identified it for what it was, nor understood that it may appear differently in different patients.

Its most common causes in the general hospital are surgery; trauma such as hip fractures; infection, especially of the lungs; medications such as opioids (meperidine, morphine, etc.), minor tranquilizers (lorazepam, diazepam, etc.), antihistamines (diphenhydramine, etc.), anticholinergics; congestive heart failure; and metabolic disturbances. The list of causes is long. Delirium is a disorder of brain function.

Let's look at some of the signs and symptoms of delirium. Delusions are false beliefs that cannot be shaken by contrary evidence or logical argument. They are common in delirium.

> Her pneumonia, heart failure, and delirium resolved, Edna McGunty apologizes to Mr. Dolbach.
> "I'm so embarrassed. Did I really spit at you. That's awful. What did you say I had?"
> "Delirium."
> "I don't ever want to have that again. It was terrifying."
> "What did you experience?"
> "I was convinced that somehow I had been removed from the hospital and taken to some basement somewhere and that I was being pumped up with drugs so they could molest me. I saw smoke. I thought I was in hell. I was trying to leave when someone came in – I think it was you – and I thought 'This is it. They're going to kill me.' I was getting up to leave. I'm so sorry. I hope I didn't hurt you."

Persecutory delusions are common in delirious patients. Whereas it makes sense to introduce yourself, speak in a reassuring tone of voice, and explain the situation, it is usually useless to try to convince the patient with persecutory delusions that she is safe. Delusions, by definition, cannot be shaken by logical evidence and argument.

Some commonly encountered delusions in delirious patients are that the nurses are having a party, even a wedding party, outside the patient's room; that the nurses are trying to kill the patient; that there is a weird conspiracy in the hospital and terrible things are going on in other rooms; that sinister strangers are impersonating nurses.

Visual hallucinations are common as well.

> Betty Mere, a previously active 65-year-old with degenerative joint disease of the spine is admitted to the hospital with a one-week history of progressive muscle weakness – Guillain-Barré. She is given morphine for pain. Within 24 hours, she

sees smoke rising from the foot of the bed and feels she's standing in bed, though she's paralyzed and supine. She is very frightened. (P.S. The morphine did it.)

John Wong, 80 years old, underwent hip replacement surgery two days ago. He begins complaining that someone's cat is loose in his room. He wants to leave the hospital immediately.

Hallucinations are false perceptions – that is, perception without a corresponding object – seeing smoke or a cat where there is none, hearing a voice when no one is speaking, smelling burnt rubber where there is none (as may occur as an aura before a temporal lobe seizure), feeling ants crawling on one's skin when there are no ants (as may occur in alcohol or benzodiazepine withdrawal), tasting chocolate where there is none. Mrs. Mere had a kinesthetic hallucination – the feeling she was standing in bed. Though hallucinations may affect all five senses, visual hallucinations are by far the most common in delirium and if a patient is having them you should assume that he is delirious.

Another characteristic of delirium is that it fluctuates in severity throughout the day.

Homer Troncos, a 65-year-old man whose course after mitral valve replacement was complicated by arrhythmias, was seen each morning by his cardiologist who found the patient oriented and appropriate, whereas the psychiatric consultant who saw him later in the day often found him confused. A CT scan of the brain revealed a cerebral infarct in the right hemisphere.

A delirious patient may look you in the eye, respond appropriately to your questions, and appear calm, only to insist, a few minutes later, on leaving the hospital for reasons you cannot understand.

How do you respond to the confused, frightened 80-year-old man, the day after hip surgery, who tells you he wants to go home "right now"? You will, of course, wish to inquire why but, whatever his reason, it is usually prudent to agree in principle with the confused, irrational patient rather that to argue with him. In this case, one might say, "Yes! We need to get you home as soon as possible," rather than saying, "You old fool, you just had a steel nail placed in your hip and you aren't going anywhere, understand." You wouldn't speak this way to a patient, of course, but imagine having other patients waiting who need dressing changes, relief from fever, analgesics, IV antibiotics, antiemetics and emesis basins, calls to the physician, etc. while your hip patient is demanding that you call a taxi.

After agreeing with the patient, you might then offer him something to eat or drink, repositioning in bed, finding a different television channel, i.e., you might attempt to divert his attention. You might wish to administer a major tranquilizer.

The general principle here is that it is usually, if not always, futile to use rational arguments with irrational people. For example, the wise parent with the child who is screaming for corn flakes when there is only oatmeal, might say, "Yes, corn flakes are delicious. Wouldn't it be great if we had some corn flakes? I'll try to get some today. How about some oatmeal until then?" rather than "No, you can't have cornflakes. Now eat your (*expletive deleted*) oatmeal" (Faber and Mazlish 1982).

Of course, it does not always make sense to agree with the patient. If a patient is frightened by visual hallucinations of bugs in the sheets you do not say, "Why yes, there are bugs in the sheets. Aren't they ugly." For one thing, "bugs in the sheets" may be a hallucination but not a delusion, i.e., the patient may "see" the bugs but not believe that there are bugs there, much as the proverbial "pink elephants" may be seen but not believed. You might wish to ask the patient if there are really bugs in the sheets or if, perhaps, his eyes are playing tricks on him. If the patient is convinced that there are bugs, i.e., is experiencing both hallucinations and delusions, you may ask his explanation for the phenomenon, how troubled he is by it. We cautiously use the phrase "may wish to" because your bedside clinical judgment must always supersede our general guidelines. It might be foolish, even dangerous, to ask the agitated patients a lot of questions rather than acting quickly to get control of the situation.

Short-term memory is inevitably impaired in delirium so that you may tell a patient in the morning that she'll be going for a chest X-ray later in the day, only to find that she is surprised and annoyed when the transporter arrives to take her to radiology. If it is important that the patient remember something, it should be repeated frequently, perhaps even be put in writing for the patient to refer to.

Not all delirious patients are agitated. Some are lethargic and somnolent. Clearly they are not as difficult to manage as are agitated patients. They are, however, frequently misidentified as suffering from a depression, rather than a delirium. Antidepressants, supportive listening, etc., will not help. The task at hand is to identify the cause of the delirium.

One of the most helpful questions in eliciting reports of hallucinations and delusions is "Did you have any unusual experiences last night?"

The agitation of delirium can be dangerous to the patient and staff. It must not be ignored. The patient may fall out of bed, dislodge an endotracheal tube, pull out an arterial or central line, bite or punch a nurse, and so forth. Except for delirium caused by alcohol or sedative hypnotic withdrawal, intravenous haloperidol is the drug of choice to calm the patient.

Haloperidol for agitation in the delirious patient

The Food and Drug Administration of the United States (FDA) has never given formal approval for the intravenous route of administration of haloperidol because no pharmaceutical firm has wished to spend the money on the formal testing that would be required for such approval. Nevertheless, there are hundreds of articles in the literature on the use of intravenous haloperidol as the drug of choice for agitation in delirium; it is universally used for this indication; and we personally have treated about a thousand delirious patients using it (Adams 1988; Riker et al. 1994; Trzepacz 1996; Gallinat et al. 1999; Centeno et al. 2004). The use of minor tranquilizers or opioids for most cases of delirium is contraindicated, usually making the delirium worse. Many nurses and physicians, however, are still reluctant to use this medication, or if they use it, use too little.

Rare complications of IV haloperidol use for agitated delirium

Some of the reasons for this reluctance, given here in no particular order, are: lack of experience with the drug and its reputation for being strong medicine; acquaintance with a psychiatric patient on haloperidol who developed tardive dyskinesia; and fear of torsade de pointes, dystonia, tardive dyskinesia, or neuroleptic malignant syndrome. Let us examine these concerns.

Lack of experience: Clearly we're more comfortable with familiar methods. The benzodiazepines may *temporarily* calm the delirious patient so that some physicians continue to order them for "agitation" which, in the general hospital, usually means "delirium". They work, however, by putting the patient to sleep and, since they seriously impair short-term memory, the patient is often more confused after he wakes up. Haloperidol had a reputation of being a potent medication and so it is avoided.

Tardive dyskinesia: Tardive is derived from the same root as tardy and means late (Glazer 2000). Dyskinesia means spasmodic or repetitive movements. This syndrome of involuntary tongue and lip movements caused by major tranquilizers develops after years of daily treatment and is not a problem in the general hospital.

Torsade de pointes, or multifocal ventricular tachycardia, is a rare problem (Sharma *et al.* 1998; Hassaballa and Balk 2003),[1] occurring in patients with preexisting cardiac disease when the QT interval is prolonged, when doses of haloperidol are "high" (100–400 mg per day), and potassium levels low. If agitation is not quickly brought under control, the much more likely danger in delirium is of falls, accidental extubations, injured nurses, prolonged hospital stays with subsequent complications such as nosocomial pneumonia, and so forth.

Most experienced nurses will have seen a few cases of acute dystonias in young patients caused by prochlorperazine. Acute dystonias caused by intravenous haloperidol in the elderly are extremely rare. Should one occur, intramuscular biperiden 5 mg or procylidine 5 mg (anticholinergics) or promethazine 50 mg or diphenhydramine 50 mg (antihistamines) are administered. We use intravenous diphenhydramine 25 mg with a second or third injection if necessary (van Harten *et al.* 1999).

Neuroleptic malignant syndrome is a rare, potentially fatal condition, caused by major tranquilizers such as haloperidol. The patient develops fever, muscular rigidity, and autonomic instability. Early recognition is vital (Susman 2001; Waldorf 2003).

Haloperidol orders

The writing of haloperidol orders is the physician's task but we include here a general description of how this should be done (Adams 1988). Depending on the severity or dangerousness of the agitation, the patient's condition, age, etc., 2 to 5 mg, sometimes 10 mg, of intravenous haloperidol is given IV push. Depending on effectiveness, the dose may be increased up to 10 mg. Administration is repeated every 30 minutes until the patient is calm. In a day or two, a routine dosing schedule is established in addition to a prn dosing. When agitation is not controlled with 10 mg of IV haloperidol given every 30 minutes, IV lorazepam may be added to the regimen, but only after each dose of IV haloperidol. Continuous intravenous haloperidol is sometimes used in the intensive care unit, with rates ranging from 5 to 50 mg per hour (Riker *et al.* 1994).

What is the maximum dose of IV haloperidol in a 24-hour period? There is no maximum dose. The decision on use is clinical, depending on the patient's response.

These patients require close observation, and should be near the nurses' station. Sometimes the presence of a family member has a calming effect. You may wish to consider letting a spouse or adult child, for example, spend the night in the room with the patient.

Making the diagnosis of delirium

You should be able to recognize delirium when you see it. The most important criterion is that there has been an acute change in cognition. This will distinguish dementia from delirium, though, of course, a patient with Alzheimer's disease may also develop a delirium. Table 8 will help you recall how the diagnosis is made and how to intervene (Burgess 1990; Antai-Otong 1995; Gonzales *et al.* 2004).

Table 8 Delirium – making the diagnosis, troubling behaviors, interventions

Making the diagnosis	Examples
• 1. Has there been a *change* in thinking, memory, or perception that came on over hours to days, i.e., an *acute* change in cognition?	• A few days ago Mr. Manley knew everyone's name but is now making mistakes. He has become forgetful, disoriented, or has developed hallucinations or delusions. You may need to ask family, friends, or other nurses if there has been an *acute* change from baseline
• 2. Does the patient have difficulty focusing *attention* or is he easily distractible?	• You have to repeat your questions because Mr. Manley's attention wanders. He can't follow the conversation. He can't, for example, say the numbers 5–9–2 backwards
• 3. Is the patient's thinking disorganized?	• Ask him why he's here. Give him a minute to answer. Disorganized means switching from subject to subject, irrelevant comments, loss of logic
• 4. Is the patient's level of consciousness altered?	• Is he, for example, hyperalert (hypervigilant) or somnolent, stuporous, or comatose?
• If you answer "yes" to both questions 1 and 2, and "yes" to either 3 or 4 you have made a diagnosis of delirium (Gonzales *et al.* 2004)	
Troubling behaviors	
• Agitation	• Mr. Manley is constantly trying to climb out of bed
• Aggression	• He threatens the nurse or strikes out at her
• Hallucinations	• He's seeing people or animals that aren't there
• Delusions	• He believes the staff is trying to hurt him
Interventions	
• If you note a new delirium assess the patient for a change in medical status.	• Is the patient developing pneumonia or a urinary tract infection, congestive heart failure, an arrhythmia, hemorrhage? Is the patient getting central nervous system depressants?
• Try verbal de-escalation	• (See Table 13)
• Use simple, direct language	
• Assume a calm, reassuring manner	
• Approach patients slowly and from the front	
• Facilitate better perception	• Get him his eyeglasses and hearing aid

continued

Table 8 (cont)

Making the diagnosis	Examples
• Move patient closer to the nurses' station if possible	
• Set limits (see Chapter 10)	
• Orient the patient	• "I'm Betty. I'm one of your nurses here at Virginia Mason Hospital."
• Use IV haloperidol or oral risperidone or olanzepine as appropriate	• Benzodiazepines, opioids, anticholinergics, and antihistamines will likely worsen cognition
• Get a sitter or use restraints if appropriate (family member, friend, or staff)	• This often reduces the need for restraints and medications but is not always possible

Table 9 Alcohol withdrawal

Stage 1a:

- The initial signs of withdrawal occur within 4 to 10 hours after the peak blood-alcohol level begins to decline
- There is tachycardia (P = 90–100)
- Systolic blood pressure increases by 10 to 20 mmHg
- Tachypnea (RR 20 to 22)
- Diaphoresis limited to the axilla
- Tremor
- Anxiety
- Increase in deep tendon reflexes

Stage 1b: 24 hours after the decline from peak blood alcohol level, there is:

- An increase in all of the above with
- Heart rate 110–120
- Systolic increase by 20–40 mm Hg
- Diaphoresis of forehead, palms, and hands
- Seizures are the hallmark of stage 1b

Three quarters or more of patients who develop stage 1 withdrawal have resolution of the syndrome in about a day, regardless of intervention.

Stage 2: or *delirium tremens*, the final phase of alcohol withdrawal:

- Usually appears 72 hours after the drop in peak blood alcohol level but may start as late as 96 or as early as 36 hours.
- Tachycardia, hypertension, tachypnea, hyperreflexia, diaphoresis, and tremor are all much increased.
- At this stage, frightening hallucinations and delusions appear and the patient may become disoriented as well.

Note
Most people have resolution of symptoms at an early stage of withdrawal; in other words, not every one progresses to stage 1b or 2.

Alcohol withdrawal and alcohol withdrawal delirium

The appearance of a patient with delirium tremens, DT's, may be indistinguishable from that of a patient with a delirium from other causes. The history and timing of the onset of signs and symptoms help make the diagnosis. The treatment of delirium tremens differs from that of delirium from other causes because here a benzodiazepine is the drug of choice. As much as 1 to 5 mg of IV lorazepam every 5 to 10 minutes may be necessary in severe cases.

Table 9 on page 42 shows one staging schema for alcohol withdrawal (Merlin 1990).

The duration of delirium

There are few studies on this question but for cases serious enough to elicit a request for help from a psychiatric consultant, about half the cases resolved in a week and half took longer (Manos and Wu 1997). No post-operative delirium lasted longer than 3 weeks but a few medically caused cases lasted a month or two.

If a patient is giving you trouble, especially an older patient, be sure he is not suffering from a delirium.

Bibliography

Adams, F. 1988 Emergency intravenous sedation of the delirious, medically ill patient. *Journal of Clinical Psychiatry*. 49:12 (Suppl.), December.

American Psychiatric Association 1994 *Diagnostic and Statistical Manual of Mental Disorders*, 4th Edn, Davis, D. C.

Antai-Otong D. 1995 *Psychiatric Nursing. Biological and Behavioral Concepts*. Philadelphia: W. B. Saunders.

Burgess AW. 1990 *Psychiatric Nursing in the Hospital and the Community*. 5th Edn. Norwalk, Ct: Appleton and Lange.

Centeno C. Sanz A. Bruera E. 2004 Delirium in advanced cancer patients. *Palliative Medicine*. 18(3):184–94, Apr.

Faber A. Mazlish E. 1982 *How to Talk so Kids will Listen and Listen so Kids Will Talk*. New York: Avon Books.

Fick DM. Agostini JV. Inouye SK. 2002 Delirium superimposed on dementia: a systematic review. *Journal of the American Geriatrics Society*. 50(10):1723–32, Oct.

Gallinat J. Moller H. Moser RL. Hegerl U. 1999 [Postoperative delirium: risk factors, prophylaxis and treatment] [German] *Anesthetist*. 48(8):507–18, Aug.

Glazer WM. 2000 Extrapyramidal side effects, tardive dyskinesia, and the concept of atypicality. *Journal of Clinical Psychiatry*. 61 (Suppl. 3):16–21.

Gonzalez M. DePablo J. Fuente E. Valdes M. Peri JM. Nomdedue M. Matrai S. 2004 Instrument for detection of delirium in general hospitals: adaptation of the confusion assessment method. *Psychosomatics*. 45(5):426–31.

Hassaballa HA. Balk RA. 2003 Torsade de pointes associated with the administration of intravenous haloperidol: a review of the literature and practical guidelines for use. *Expert Opinion on Drug Safety*. 2(6):543–7, Nov.

Kolbeinsson H. Jonsson A. 1993 Delirium and dementia in acute medical admissions of elderly patients in Iceland. *Acta Psychiatrica Scandinavica*. 87(2):123–7, Feb.

Lechin F. van der Dijs B. Benaim M. 1996 Benzodiazepines: tolerability in elderly patients. *Psychotherapy & Psychosomatics*. 65(4):171–82.

Manos PJ. Wu R. 1997 The duration of delirium in medical and postoperative patients referred for psychiatric consultation. *Annals of Clinical Psychiatry.* 9(4): 219–26.

Merlin SI. 1990 Treatment of the alcohol withdrawal syndrome. In *Hospital Based Treatment of Substance Abuse.* Chapter 7. WM Lerner, Ed. NY: Plenum Press.

Riker RR. Fraser GL. Cox PM. 1994 Continuous infusion of haloperidol controls agitation in critically ill patients. *Critical Care Medicine* 22(3):433–9.

Rockwood K. 1993 The occurrence and duration of symptoms in elderly patients with delirium. *Journal of Gerontology.* 48(4):M162–6, Jul.

Sharma ND. Rosman HS. Padhi ID. Tisdale JE. 1998 Torsades de pointes associated with intravenous haloperidol in critically ill patients. *American Journal of Cardiology.* 81(2):238–40, Jan 15.

Susman VL. 2001 Clinical management of neuroleptic malignant syndrome. *Psychiatric Quarterly.* 72(4):325–36, Winter.

Trzepacz PT. 1996 Delirium. Advances in diagnosis, pathophysiology, and treatment. *Psychiatric Clinics of North America.* 19(3):429–48, Sep.

van der Mast RC. 2003 [The Dutch College of General Practitioners' practice guideline 'Delirium in elderly people'; response from psychiatry]. [Dutch] *Nederlands Tijdschrift voor Geneeskunde.* 147(20):952–5, May 17.

van Harten PN. Hoek HW. Kahn RS. 1999 Acute dystonia induced by drug treatment. *British Medical Journal.* 319(7210):623–6, Sep 4.

Waldorf S. 2003 AANA journal course. Update for nurse anesthetists. Neuroleptic malignant syndrome. *AANA Journal.* 71(5):389–94, Oct.

Webster R. Holroyd S. 2000 Prevalence of psychotic symptoms in delirium. *Psychosomatics.* 41(6):519–22, Nov–Dec.

Chapter 4

Psychiatric diagnoses

Nursing students may be intimidated when assigned a patient with a psychiatric diagnosis, the formidable patient referred to in whispers as "the psych patient". We hope here to demystify the diagnoses by describing some of the symptoms and behaviors patients *may* exhibit. We will not review the course of these conditions, how diagnoses are made, or prevalence, which can be found in standard texts including DSM IV (American Psychiatric Association 1994) from which much of the following is paraphrased.

Mania as seen in bipolar affective disorder (manic depressive illness)

Denise Rappinet, a 54-year-old aircraft mechanic and mother of two, fractured a metacarpal and severely cut her arm when she punched her fist through the kitchen window of her eldest son's home after they had quarreled. She was seen in the emergency room and sent directly to surgery. The operation required vascular reconstruction and the patient was admitted to the hospital for observation. Don Dolbach, R.N., was assigned to her care. The day after surgery she appeared in remarkably good spirits despite some swelling of the arm and was appreciative of her nurse's attention.

"That was painless. You changed that dressing like a professional."

"I am a professional."

They laughed together and rapport seemed solid.

During the day, she put on her own clothes and began visiting other patients in their rooms spreading good cheer. When the surgeon came by to inspect her wound she was nowhere to be found. He came back later but she was still absent. Annoyed, he wrote an order for her to stay in her room until he could examine the wound. When she reappeared, Mr. Dolbach explained the situation.

"But I can't just stay in here. My blood pressure is already high and if I can't walk around, I'm afraid I'll have a stroke."

He measured her blood pressure, which was fine, and reassured her.

"You are such a good nurse and I am relieved. But I'm afraid I'm going to start worrying about it anyway unless I can walk around. Then I'll have to call you every fifteen minutes to check it, which is totally unreasonable. I promise I will stay on the floor and will not go into anyone's room. I'll be visible. I just can't sit here waiting for Dr. Jones the whole time."

"You're going to stay on the floor."

"Absolutely."

"Alright."

"Don, you're a prince."

She was not only absent from the floor when Dr. Jones returned, she was away all night.

The next day, disheveled, wet, her bandage unraveling, she explained that a frail old man had appeared about to fall so she helped him onto the elevator and walked him to the front of the hospital. When his ride didn't arrive, she called a cab and escorted him home. He paid the fare.

She had no funds to get back to the hospital so she hitchhiked back in the rain. Mr. Dolbach, having already been embarrassed in front of the doctor when the patient was missing overnight, was now furious that the wound might be compromised. Mrs. Rappinet wondered how she could possibly be blamed for trying to help out a poor old man in need. Didn't the nurse have a heart? Perhaps she'd misjudged him. When he asked to check the wound, she refused, and walked to the nurses' station.

"I've just had a terrible night and I need some compassion. Is there someone who can check my wound? That man is just too rough."

Bipolar affective disorder, also know as manic-depressive illness, is a serious disorder of mood regulation, involving periods of depression and periods of mania. The symptoms and behaviors likely to be most disturbing for the nursing staff of a general hospital occur during mania (Goodwin and Jamison 1990; Jamison 1995).

Mania is a persistently elevated, expansive, or irritable mood of such intensity that it markedly impairs occupational or social functioning. Mrs. Rappinet's case illustrates this.

The elevated mood may be described as euphoric, elated, unusually good, cheerful, or high. Friends or relatives recognize that the patient is not her usual self, but those unfamiliar with her may initially find the patient charming and delightful, at least for a while.

The patient may unceasingly and indiscriminately seek interpersonal, sexual, or occupational interactions, drawing strangers into conversation, flirting, or making long distance phone calls.

Mood may be irritable instead of expansive, so that the patient may become angry and demanding when her wishes are not met.

Self-esteem may be so inflated that the patient may believe she has a special relationship with God, the president, or some other public figure. With no prior experience, she may embark on writing a novel, obtaining patents for unrealistic ideas or inventions, giving investment advice to experts in the field.

Manic speech is loud, rapid, and difficult to interrupt. It may be amusing to listen to with puns, jokes, and theatrical flourishes. If the mood is irritable rather than euphoric the patient may go on angry tirades.

It is unlikely that the patient with bipolar illness will be in an acute manic phase during a stay in a general hospital, but if the patient is manic, the nurse should be aware of some of the difficulty dealing with her.

The acutely manic patient is difficult to deal with in any setting, no less so in the setting of the general hospital (Janoswsky *et al.* 1970). Because the bright, cheerful, entertaining, and euphoric patient may genuinely, albeit transiently, feel that the nurse caring for her is wonderful, the nurse himself may experience inflated self-esteem. He may become invested in maintaining that inflated self-esteem. But later when her wishes are thwarted, the patient may turn on the nurse, with unusual perceptiveness about the nurse's areas of personal vulnerability, putting the nurse on the defensive, making him more worried about his own self-esteem than the patient's well-being.

Manic patients are exceptionally good at selling an idea and making an excuse. Because the manic patient is so sure of herself, so unambivalent, her illogical reasoning may sound reasonable. The simplest thing to remember about caring for such patients is to set limits, even if the patient argues that they are arbitrary, and stick to them. Note also that sometimes high dose steroids can set off a hypomanic or manic episode.

Schizophrenia

> Bill Tweedy, a 24-year-old admitted with appendicitis, is seen the day after surgery by Don Dolbach, R.N.
> "Do you think I'm going to be alright?"
> "Of course, you are. You came through surgery with flying colors. Your fever is way down. Don't you feel well?"
> "They took out my appendix."
> "Yes, it was infected."
> "Can I see it?"
> "Well, I don't think so. They've disposed of it."
> "How do they know it was infected?"
> "The pathologist examined it."
> "What does the pathologist look like?"
> "I don't know the pathologist."
> "But you work here, don't you?"
> "Yes, of course I work here, and I know your appendix was inflamed and could have killed you if it hadn't been removed."
> "But they're saying I'm a fool."
> "I don't understand. Who's saying you're a fool?"
> "They are. The voices. They said my appendix wasn't removed and it wasn't infected."
> "Well, it was. Ask the doctor . . . Are you hearing the voices now?"
> "Yes."
> "What are they saying?"
> "That I'm a fool."
> "Are they telling you to do anything or to hurt yourself?"
> "No. Don't you think I have a right to see my appendix?"
> "I think you should talk with the doctor about that."

Schizophrenia is really not one, but rather a group of mental illnesses with different biochemical and neurological etiologies, which, at this time in medical understanding, are included under one heading. Patients with these disorders may misinterpret and retreat from reality, thinking and acting erratically, bizarrely, or angrily. However, those receiving appropriate treatment may seem no different than any other patient (Torrey 2001).

The first psychotic episode of schizophrenia usually begins in the early or mid-twenties for men, the late twenties for women, though prodromal symptoms may have been present for years. During such an acute episode and to some degree during the entire course of the illness, both positive and negative symptoms may be present. Positive symptoms may include delusions, hallucinations, disorganized speech, and disorganized or catatonic behavior. Negative symptoms include affective flattening, paucity of thought and speech, and the inability to initiate action.

Delusions – fixed, false beliefs that cannot be shaken by incontrovertible evidence – are found in several disorders, but are particularly common in schizophrenia. The most common theme is of persecution: being spied on, tricked, followed, ridiculed, and plotted against. Also common are delusions of reference, the belief that ideas, instructions, messages etc. are specifically being directed at the person through the TV, radio, passages in newspapers and books, or through the gestures of people around the patient, or even through the way the bed has been made or food arranged on the dinner tray.

Although occurring in other conditions, bizarre delusions are most often associated with schizophrenia. The belief that one's organs have been replaced by someone else's, that one is being controlled by radio waves transmitted by aliens, that one's thoughts have been removed by an outside force, or that thoughts have been put into one's head by an outside force – all these are considered bizarre. The delusion that one is under surveillance by the police is considered non-bizarre.

Hallucinations are most commonly auditory: a voice talking about the person, or two or more voices speaking with each other about the person, usually in a derogatory way. Visual hallucinations are rare and if present suggest a problem such as delirium, not schizophrenia.

Speech may be disorganized, so that a person moves from one topic to another without an obvious association between successive topics; answers may only be obliquely related to questions; or speech may be incomprehensible (word salad).

Disorganized behavior may include childlike silliness, unpredictable outbursts of shouting or strange gesticulation, inability to maintain hygiene, bizarre dress.

The person may show facial immobility, poor eye contact and unresponsiveness, utter brief, empty replies, and simply sit for long periods.

This description of symptoms of acute and chronic decompensation in this devastating illness make clear why a flagrantly psychotic patient may frighten the experienced as well as the inexperienced. The first order of business is to assess the safety of the patient and the safety of the staff.

How do you ask the patient if he is having delusions? Since the most common theme is persecutory, you can ask the patient, "Has anybody been against you, been giving you a hard time, or accusing you of things?" "Are people too critical of you?"

To assess hallucinations, "Do you hear voices that others can't hear?" "What are they saying?" "Are they telling you to do something?"

Other questions to ask or consider asking: "Do you feel safe here?" "Do you feel a need to defend yourself?" "Are you thinking about hurting someone or getting even?" "Are you thinking about hurting yourself?"

Since most of the patients with schizophrenia in the general hospital will already have had their symptoms brought under control with major tranquilizers, you should not assume, before actually seeing the patient, that these symptoms will be present. The patient may, in fact, be indistinguishable in this respect from all your other patients. Remember it is usually the person who becomes difficult, not the diagnosis.

Somatoform disorders

Consider two patients of whom you know nothing but the following:

> Both Ms. Abbott and Ms. Bishop have had major medical work-ups, negative to date, for symptoms that seriously affect their day-to-day lives.
>
> Ms. Abbott to her doctor, "You know, Dr. Pope, I know I've been sick but I'm wondering if maybe it's depression or something. I'm having problems with my husband and my 16-year-old son. I'm under considerable stress. Could that be causing my problems?"
>
> Ms. Bishop to her doctor, "I've already told you there is no stress in my life. My husband and children are wonderful. I'm just sick all the time. That's the only stress. Maybe I need an operation, Dr. Pope. I've probably got cancer or something."

One of these patients has pancreatic cancer. The other has a somatoform disorder, a condition with symptoms out of proportion to any physical findings or diagnosable medical problem, though the symptoms suggest the presence of a physical illness. We will discuss only three somatoform disorders: somatization disorder (Briquet's syndrome), conversion disorder, and somatoform pain disorder (Ford 1983).

Most patients with *somatization disorder* are women. The problem begins before age thirty. Patients complain of pain and of multiple, diverse disturbances involving the gastrointestinal, reproductive, and nervous systems. They may seek care from multiple providers, often undergoing invasive diagnostic procedures and surgery.

You may see these patients when they are admitted to the hospital for symptomatic treatment (control of pain, nausea and vomiting, pseudoneurological symptoms) or for further diagnostic work-up before the diagnosis has been made.

These patients are not necessarily difficult to work with since they have achieved what they want, namely medical attention. A few points to remember: although their description of their problem is often dramatic and vague, their distress is real: they are not pretending to be ill (compare with factitious illness).

In *conversion disorder* the patient has unexplained symptoms involving motor or sensory function: paralysis, weakness, even blindness. These pseudoneurological symptoms may also be seen in somatization disorder. Psychological factors are judged to be associated with the symptoms.

In *somatoform pain disorder* complaints of pain are predominant and psychological factors have an important role in the onset, severity, or maintenance of the condition.

All these disorders suggest a disturbance in the body, the soma, hence the name, somatoform. Even when thorough medical evaluation fails to reveal a cause, these patients are reluctant even to consider the role that past or current stress plays in their illness. That is, they are not psychologically minded. They do not recognize their emotional distress though it may be intense. Instead it is expressed in the body with pain, nausea, fatigue, weakness, paralysis, sexual dysfunction, etc. Some patients with somatoform disorder do indeed have medical problems, but symptoms are grossly out of proportion to what would be expected based on the nature of the problem and on the physical findings.

Mrs. Abbott is psychologically minded. She has cancer. Mrs. Bishop is unaware of the stress in her life and instead develops bodily complaints. She has a somatoform disorder.

Factitious disorder

Mrs. Bishop is not pretending to be ill; rather her occult emotional distress is converted unconsciously into somatic symptoms. Patients with factitious disorders, on the other hand, *are* pretending to be ill. Signs and symptoms are intentionally produced or feigned in order to attain the sick role. No other reasonable motive can be identified.

These patients are not malingering, that is, they are not pretending to be ill in order to avoid conscription, trial, or jail, or to obtain money, food, drugs, or a bed for the night. When a malingerer's situation is known, then the motive for "illness" is clear. Not so for the patient with factitious illness. All the factitious patient wants is the sick role.

Suspicion of this disorder is raised when the patient's presentation is atypical or dramatic, not conforming to an identifiable psychiatric or medical disorder; when behaviors are present only when the patient knows he is being observed; when he is disruptive on the ward, arguing with nurses and doctors, breaking hospital rules; when he has extensive knowledge of medical terminology and hospital routine; when he surreptitiously uses drugs; when he has traveled extensively; when complications develop rapidly as soon as the initial work-up is negative; when pseudologia fantastica is present – pathological lying intriguing to the listener, i.e., tall tales.

Psychopathological disease simulation, i.e., factitious illness, shows a spectrum of severity (Nadelson 1979). Some non-prototypical patients (often nurses), are working, infrequently producing illness (Guziec *et al*. 1994). Others spend their whole lives getting admitted to hospitals – Münchausen's syndrome, after Baron von Münchausen who traveled widely and told dramatic stories (Sutherland and Rodin 1990; Wise and Ford 1999).

We quote from Richard Asher's 1951 original description of the syndrome. "Often the diagnosis is made by a passing doctor or sister, who, recognizing the patient and his performance, exclaims, 'I know this man. We had him in St. Quinidine's two years ago and thought he had a perforated ulcer. He's the man who always collapses on buses and tells a story about being an ex-submarine commander who was tortured by the Gestapo.'"

When confronted and narcotic analgesics withdrawn, these patients often leave the hospital against medical advice.

An even more troubling syndrome is Münchausen's syndrome by proxy in which one person, often the mother of a child, inflicts on another person, often her child, the stigmata of illness, and repeatedly seeks care for the "patient" (Moldavsky and Stein 2002).

Personality disorders

A personality disorder is an enduring pattern of maladaptive behavior, beginning in adolescence, which leads to distress or impairment. The following personality disorders are described in DSM IV: paranoid, schizoid, schizotypal, antisocial, borderline, histrionic, narcissistic, avoidant, dependent, obsessive-compulsive, and personality disorder not otherwise specified (Millon 1995). Here we briefly discuss only two.

Antisocial personality disorder

Persons with *antisocial personality disorder* disregard and violate the rights of others, using deceit and manipulation to obtain personal profit or pleasure. They may repeatedly harass others, destroy property, steal, or engage in other crimes. They may be superficially charming and glib. The caveats with such persons are: maintain vigilance for manipulation, communicate with your colleagues, and set limits.

Martin Score, a handsome, well-built man tattooed with the names of five different women and five different states, presents to the emergency room explaining that he had an accident while working for a construction company in Indonesia and now, on a long return flight home, has developed excruciating chest pain that he fears may be a pulmonary embolism.

He is admitted and continues to complain bitterly of unrelieved pain demanding higher and higher does of morphine on the patient-controlled analgesia machine. He often goes out to smoke.

Mr. Score is angry and impulsive, frightening the patient in the next bed, the transporter, and another nurse on the floor, but he enthralls Dr. Marsh, the intern, with tales of his work as a Navy SEAL and Ms. Jones, his primary nurse, a recent nursing school graduate, with the story of how he cared for his dying wife. He's planning to buy a house in town, settle down, and marry a woman who already has children. It so happens Ms. Jones meets this profile. Captivated, she makes a special effort to attend to his needs (*see also boundary violations*).

He refuses to have a pulmonary angiogram but insists on ever increasing doses of morphine. Finally he suffers a respiratory arrest, quickly reversed with Narcan. On awakening, he's light-hearted and wants to go down for a smoke. Ms. Davis, an experienced supervising nurse, insists that the patient be confined to the floor immediately after resuscitation, lest the Narcan wear off and he suffer another respiratory arrest. The intern yields but tells Ms. Davis not to make the patient feel bad.

All along the supervising nurse has futilely tried to get the primary nurse and the intern to set limits, pointing out the inconsistencies in Mr. Score's story and his disruptive behavior. Dr. Marsh explains to Ms. Davis that Navy SEALs learn to lie in order to survive. The primary nurse and intern feel that her attempts at limit setting are excessive, possibly even vindictive.

Mr. Score has also been pressing to have a peripherally inserted central catheter (PICC) placed for blood drawing. Ms. Davis points out to the intern the clear inappropriateness of this, to which he concedes. Later, he and the primary nurse console and commiserate with the patient.

Mr. Score tries to file a quality assurance complaint against Ms. Davis claiming that she's mistreating him, but the hospital quality assurance office can find no grounds for his claim.

During trips out to smoke, he strikes up conversations with various patients and staff members, his charm undeniable. A clerk from another unit of the hospital begins visiting him. After a while, though she has no direct experience of the patient's interactions with the supervising nurse, she goes to the quality assurance office to confirm the patient's complaints. The office now opens a case. The patient also makes clear that he plans to file a complaint with the state board of licensing.

Finally the patient consents to a pulmonary angiogram. There is no pulmonary embolus. On returning to his room Mr. Score pulls out his IV line and throws a chair against the wall. He's also furious that he didn't get a PICC line. He leaves AMA.

A few days later the clerk who had befriended him goes to the quality assurance office to retract her complaint. It appears that Mr. Score has taken her credit card and disappeared with her new car after taking it for "test drive".

All along the supervising nurse had expressed her concerns and given guidance, only to have her reputation and her nurse's license threatened. When the havoc was over, though aggrieved at the feeling of abandonment she had experienced, she methodically met with staff members to help clarify what had happened and mend the damage. Had this particular sociopath not stolen the car and credit card, permanent hard feeling among the staff might have remained.[1] We are all susceptible to charm and flattery.

Borderline personality disorder

No matter how well we may be prepared some patients will still cause havoc in the general hospital. Among these, patients with borderline personality may be the most troublesome. James Groves's chapter on *borderline personality disorders* is the basis for the following discussion (Groves 1987).

The adjective "borderline" was initially chosen in the naming of this syndrome because these patients are so unstable in interpersonal relationships, self-image, and mood, that they were felt to be on the border between neurotic suffering and psychosis (loss of touch with reality). They may polarize staff, act violently, refuse treatment, or threaten to leave against medical advice or to commit suicide. They may be impulsive and angry.

Often times, the diagnosis has not been made, but the nurse may sense a disturbance in the way a patient behaves and responds to others. Personality disorder diagnoses are notoriously difficult to make and it is not for the nurse to try to do so, nevertheless we believe it may be of help for the nurse to understand in general the criteria for such a diagnosis.

A person may have a borderline personality if he or she has had life-long instability in self-image, interpersonal relationships, and mood and meets five of the following nine criteria:

- Impulsiveness
- Moodiness
- Paranoia or dissociation under stress
- Unstable self-image
- Labile intense interpersonal relationships
- Suicidal gestures
- Inappropriate anger
- Vulnerability to abandonment, and
- Emptiness.

The mnemonic is "IMPULSIVE" and the following questions address each item in order (Senger 1995):

- Are you by nature an impulsive person?
- Are you moody?
- Do you tend to get very suspicious of people or go to pieces under stress?
- Do you often wonder who you are, what you want, or what you ought to do?
- Are your relationships with people unstable, stormy, or on-again off-again?
- Do you do self-damaging things like scratch your wrist or take too many pills?
- Do you have a temper and lose control of your anger very easily?
- Are you sensitive to rejection and easily feel abandoned?
- Do you often feel empty inside?

Much of what we now have to say about the management of these patients is covered in other sections of the book, but some learning occurs through repetition so we will repeat ourselves. Keep in mind also that though patients may carry the same diagnosis they are still individuals and can be expected to act differently from one another.

We will review several aspects of behavior that are particularly troubling for staff.

First, is a misperception of reality, but not necessarily full-blown delusional thinking. We have often talked about not confronting the frankly delusional patient, but often with borderline personality disorder, the patient must be confronted with reality as this illustration from Dr. Grove's chapter illustrates:

Patient: I don't trust you.
Consultant: Why should you – you've never seen me before. I'm Dr. Smith. Dr. Jones asked me to help you with your anxiety.
Patient: Dr. Jones hates me.
Consultant: Dr. Jones is irritated with your pulling out your intravenous tubing, but he isn't going to harm you.
Patient: You're like all of them – want to kill a guy.
Consultant: You're wrong about that. We want to help you get over this infection.
Patient: Bullshit!
Consultant: No bullshit.

Patients with borderline personality disorders may wish both to be close to other people but also fear closeness, explaining, in part, why their relationships are on-again off-again. Fear of treatment and inability to trust, coupled with inadequate ways of managing fear, a poor self-image, and a sense of entitlement may lead to denial of reality in the medical setting. The staff must appeal to the patient's sense of entitlement and try to use wording that the patient – exquisitely attuned to denigrating nuances – will not interpret as degrading. They are dependent and use manipulation – intense, covert, and often self-defeating – to get their needs met. Dr. Groves provides another illustration.

Consultant: Now what is this about your not taking the antibiotics that Dr. Black has prescribed?

Patient: I am not going to talk especially with that one here. Listen, I don't like her face and you can't force me, force this crap down my throat!

Consultant: Well, you don't have to like this lady here, and there's no particular reason why you should have to like me either, but there are several very good reasons why you should take your antibiotics that Dr. Black prescribed for you.

Patient: Yeah, well, I'm not going to take that damn stuff. Get me a lawyer! I know my rights!

Consultant: You have every right to the best medical care we can give you. Why is it that you feel so strongly against the antibiotics that Dr. Black has prescribed for you?

Patient: It's no good and, besides, Dr. Green said I oughtn't ever take antibiotics.

Consultant: Dr Green said you should never take antibiotics? Really?

Patient: He said they'd kill me.

Consultant: Really? How come?

Patient [*shouts*]: Are you saying that Dr. Green is a liar?!

[*Realizing he has stimulated the patient's rage, and been pitted against Dr. Green, the consultant returns to an appeal to the patient's entitlement*]

Consultant: Dr. Green . . . was he your doctor from before?

Patient: Best damn doctor I ever had and one million times better than the rest of you put together!

Consultant: Sounds like you like him a lot. He saw you through that other time you were in the hospital.

Patient: Yes.

Consultant: And at that time you didn't need antibiotics.

Patient: Listen, goddammit, I am not going to take that crap!

Consultant: Well, the reason I ask is that you now have a fever from this infection and we on the staff feel that you deserve to have it treated in the best way possible.

Patient: Dr. Black, what does she know?

Consultant: Well, we all feel. . . .

Patient:	I am not . . . look, Dr. Green said that I shouldn't take antibiotics.
Consultant:	. . . that you deserve the best possible treatment of this infection. I'm sure that if Dr. Green were here now he would want you to have the very best possible treatment of this infection, that he would agree that you deserve . . .
Patient:	Well get him here. Get him on the phone.
Consultant:	I can't. [*pauses*] Don't you think that if Dr. Green knew you were suffering from an infection that he would want you to have antibiotics, that he would want you to get the very best treatment, which you deserve.
Patient:	No.
Consultant:	You don't feel you deserve the best possible care of this infection?
Patient:	Get her out of here! I don't like her face.
Consultant:	We're going to leave you now for a little while and I hope that you'll think it over and allow yourself to have the kind of good medical care you're entitled to.

These appeals to the patient's sense of entitlement must be repeated. Although in these examples it is a psychiatric consultant making the appeals, we believe that it is the attending physician who should make them first, followed by the nursing staff and others.

As clinicians, we must all be aware of the sadistic urges engendered in us by such manipulative, dependent patients. Being aware of them, we can harmlessly and perhaps even amusingly express them verbally among ourselves. They must not be expressed in any way with our patients. Maintaining a civil tone of voice and choosing words that will not stoke an angry fire, we can still talk honestly with patients about our frustrations, when and if this seems appropriate.

Awareness of sadistic urges in caregivers may actually inhibit them from appropriate limit setting. Remember limit setting is to protect the patient and the staff. Doubtless some patients will accuse the setter of limits as punishing him, so it should be clear that it is not the person delivering the message but the entire staff that believes limits must be set.

Anorexia nervosa

The features of anorexia nervosa are refusal to maintain a minimally normal body weight, intense fear of gaining weight, and a disturbed body image. Patients with this disorder often lack insight, deny the problem, and are unreliable historians. Reliable outside sources of information are often necessary to get a complete picture of the problem. The most common difficulty for nurses with these patients is, of course, that the patients are in the hospital for malnutrition, but don't want anything that will cause weight gain. Their management, as with many difficult patients, demands a unified, consistent, team approach (Maxmen *et al.* 1974; Brownell and Fairburn 1995).

Concluding remarks

Familiarity with the signs and symptoms of psychiatric disorders should not only lessen anxiety, but increase clinical acumen and effectiveness as well. The nurse's focus in caring for these patients in the general hospital is primarily their medical and surgical conditions, not their psychiatric condition. These patients are just as appreciative of good care as are other patients.

Bibliography

Asher R. Munchausen's syndrome. 1951 *The Lancet* i:339–41.

Brownell KD. Fairburn CG. Eds 1995 *Eating Disorders and Obesity. A Comprehensive Handbook*. New York: The Guilford Press.

Cleckly HM. 1964 *The Mask of Sanity*. 4th Edn. St. Louis: Mosby Medical.

Ford CV. 1983 *The Somatizing Disorder. Illness as a way of life*. New York: Elsevier Biomedical.

Goodwin FK. Jamison KR. 1990 *Manic-depressive Illness*. New York: Oxford University Press.

Groves J. 1987 Borderline patients. In *Massachusetts General Hospital Handbook of General Hospital Psychiatry*. Littleton, Mass.: PSG Publishing Company, Inc.

Guziec J. Lazarus A. Harding JJ. 1994 Case of a 29-year-old nurse with factitious disorder. The utility of psychiatric intervention on a general medical floor. *General Hospital Psychiatry*. 16(1):47–53, Jan.

Jamison KR. 1995 *An Unquiet Mind*. New York: Vintage Books.

Janoswsky DS. Leff M. Epstein RS. 1970 Playing the manic game. Interpersonal maneuvers of the acutely manic patient. *Archives of General Psychiatry*. 22:252–61.

Linehan M. 1993 *Cognitive-Behavioral Treatment of Borderline Personality*. New York: The Guilford Press.

Maxmen JS. Siberfarb PM. Ferrell RB. 1974 Anorexia nervosa. Practical initial management in a general hospital. *JAMA*. 229(7):801–3, Aug 12.

Millon T. 1995. *Disorders of Personality: DSM IV and Beyond*. 2nd Edn. Canada: John Wiley and Sons.

Minuchin S. Rosman BL. Baker L. 1978 *Psychosomatic Families: Anorexia Nervosa in Context*. Cambridge, Mass.: Harvard University Press.

Moldavsky M. Stein D. 2002 Munchausen Syndrome by Proxy: two case reports and an update of the literature. *International Journal of Psychiatry in Medicine*. 33(4):411–23.

Nadelson T. 1979 The Munchausen spectrum. Borderline character features. *General Hospital Psychiatry*. 1:11–17.

Senger HL. 1995 Borderline mnemonic. [Letter] *American Journal of Psychiatry*. 36(2):1321.

Sutherland AJ. Rodin GM. 1990 Factitious disorders in a general hospital setting: clinical features and a review of the literature. *Psychosomatics*. 31(4):392–9, Fall.

Torrey EF. 2001 *Surviving Schizophrenia: A Manual for Families, Consumers, and Providers*. New York: HarperCollins.

Wise MG. Ford CV. 1999 Factitious disorders. *Primary Care; Clinics in Office Practice*. 26(2):315–26, Jun.

Chapter 5

Setting limits

All natural phenomena have limits, demarcations beyond which there is no going further. Even the universe extends only so far, has only so many galaxies, is only so old. There are limits on the subatomic scale, too, nothing shorter than the Planck length, for example, a very short distance. There are also man-made limits – speed limits, age limits, legal limits. Unlike natural limits, these can be exceeded but at some risk.

In the hospital, often the nurse must clarify for patients the limits of behavior and enforce those limits. Nurses are unprepared to do this. They did not see police work in their future, nor would have a palm reader, except for the rare palm reader with 25 years of general nursing experience. It is, of course, usually only the exceptional patient who needs such limit setting and limit enforcement.

Setting limits is often natural and unproblematic. Urinating on the floor; climbing out of bed immediately after femoral vein catheterization; smoking in bed; fiddling with the patient-controlled analgesia (PCA) machine; spitting out one's pills; pulling out one's nasogastric tube, IV line, endotracheal tube or Foley catheter, are clearly impermissible. The nurse will waste no time wondering if the patient should be allowed to do these things.

Depending on the patient's cognitive and emotional status, limit setting may range from a cheerful, "Please don't do that" to calling for urgent assistance, holding the patient down, and medicating with haloperidol. Such limit setting is generally not emotionally taxing because unequivocal danger to the patient demands that the nurse act. Better a little patient irritation now, than a lot of patient bleeding later. Soul searching is unnecessary.

Consider the following, however. What is the limit on the number of times a patient should use the call light each hour? On the number of requests a day for opioid analgesics? On the number of visitors in the room? On the number of f-words used per shift? On the time off the floor for a smoke? On the time it takes to get from bed to commode with assistance? On refusals to allow blood pressure to be measured? On refusals to work with the physical therapist? On the time it takes to get out of bed? On the volume of a patient's voice?

What is unreasonable and reasonable, i.e., what the limits should and shouldn't be is no longer a simple matter. The limits must be decided by the nurse individually or by the nursing staff collectively. Many factors are at play – the ward tolerance for the behavior, the danger of the behavior itself, the patient's condition, etc.

Setting limits means the deliberate demarcation by the nurse for the patient of a line that may not be crossed. The line is always one of behavior – either the patient's or the nurse's. In other words, the nurse may prohibit the patient from swearing at her or smoking in the bathroom or she may explain her limits, that, for example, she will not call the doctor again, or give the morphine injection before it is scheduled.

Sometimes, as part of setting limits, the nurse will also explain to the patient the consequences of crossing the line – that she'll have to call her supervisor or the attending physician, for example, if the swearing or smoking continues. The confused patient, however, is unlikely to benefit from explanations. Enforcement of limits will be accomplished by other means – getting a sitter, calling security, applying restraints, sedating the patient, calling for psychiatric consultation, and so forth.

The first obstacle to effective limit setting may be in the nurse.

> Mr. T, a 24-year-old diabetic man who wishes to be called Bobby, admitted to the hospital with ketoacidosis as the result of poor self-care, continually calls for the nurse to get him things from his bedside table – a book, water, the telephone, etc., or to adjust his bed up or down. Yet these things are within reach and he is able to do them himself. The nurse responds but becomes increasingly irritated at the squandering of her time and so takes longer and longer before entering his room. Bob's behavior deteriorates further.

This kind of problem begins insidiously. The patient asks that a glass of water be poured from the pitcher. Happy to see the patient has started drinking, the nurse responds. One request leads to many others. Unsure what to do about this and concerned about the patient's reaction should she say anything about it, she continues responding to requests.

Ah, but this is an easy one, you say, and, in fact, it is. The nurse need only control her irritation and gently tell the patient, "Bobby, you should reach for that book yourself. It'll be good for your recovery if you start doing as much for yourself as possible." Of course, the earlier said, the better.

Some patients use this tactic to have a nurse with them as much as possible because they are frightened or lonely. Or they may continually call to report a new twinge of pain, sense of nausea, sense of warmth, inability to get comfortable, or to request medication, or to ask a question, etc. Until the nurse knows this patient, each complaint will be carefully evaluated. Finally, when it becomes clear that the patient simply wants the nurse there all the time, irritation sets in – either at the system for not allowing more time with patients or at the patient himself. This is not the place for a critique of ever lower nurse to patient ratios in the hospital nor would such a critique necessarily be relevant, since this sort of patient is taxing in any system. Nor should it be necessary for us to express the sadness evoked in all of us by the sick, frightened, and lonely patient. Whatever our emotional response here, something must be done.

The above scenarios are so common that you may already do the following. After assuring yourself that the patient is stable, if needy, you tell him, "I want to keep a careful eye on you so I'm going to come by every half hour. You don't need to call me because I'm coming anyway." After that you must, of course, go by every half hour but the time spent can and should be brief – perhaps a pulse check, a fluffing of the pillow, a comforting word, or maybe just a peek in the room to ask if everything's okay – and zip out the door with the words, "I'll be back soon." Though total time spent with the patient per shift may decrease, patient satisfaction may increase because of more frequent visits.

Because some patients complain so bitterly, acting as if they are being punished, the nurse, believing that setting limits is cruel, may feel guilty. The nurse may simply wish to avoid the conflict that setting limits may produce. Nevertheless, limit setting is meant foremost to be in the patient's best interest. Even reducing the number of unnecessary calls for the nurse is in the patient's best interest because the patient is no longer avoided, hence receives better care.

Some limit setting is often best done with the physician, especially regarding medication orders. As we discuss in the chapter on substance abuse, it is often best to treat patients with routinely scheduled narcotic analgesics rather than with prn medications. The dose of medication should be adequate to treat pain and the drug dependent patient will probably need higher doses of narcotic analgesics than the average patient. Together the nurse and physician should set appropriate limits.

Mrs. G., a 58-year-old heavy-set government clerk, previously a striptease dancer, had years ago undergone a jejunoileal bypass for obesity and then a bowel resection because of bleeding. She developed a short bowel syndrome, hyperoxaluria, and consequent renal failure. Admitted to the hospital with calciphylaxis and paniculitis, she screamed continuously during dressing changes, though she had been doing them herself before admission. Though they were ordered as wet to dry, she insisted the bandages be moistened before removal, defeating their purpose – debridement. The nursing staff was greatly stressed by Mrs. G.'s screaming and demands that dressing changes be done extremely slowly.

Mrs. G. insisted on laying fully naked in bed, saying alternately either that it was too hot in the room or that the sheets were painful to her. Her nudity was distressing to the many different staff members who had to enter the room – dietitians, physical therapists, physicians, nurses, custodians, etc. – yet she wanted staff members to spend long periods of time with her.

She requested and received large doses of narcotic analgesics around the clock and prior to dressing changes as well.

As you might expect, Mrs. G. evoked strong feelings in the nursing staff. Some thought of the patient purely as a poor soul and tried to protect her or meet her wishes; others, while acknowledging the pathos of the patient's situation, nevertheless felt she was grossly inappropriate and manipulative; still others simply wanted to avoid her because she was too demanding. Because Mrs. G. responded to attempts at limit setting as if she were being punished, some nurses felt that limit setting was indeed punishment. They felt that all her requests for narcotic analgesics were justified. The patient added to this split perspective of the staff, by praising some nurses – those who did as she asked – and vilifying others – those who did not always do as she asked. So disruptive was this patient's behavior and personality that several very good nurses began eyeing each other with mistrust, if not antagonism.

After four months of continuous hospitalization, a psychiatric consultation was asked for. Why it took so long is unclear, but by the time the consultant was involved, the normally effective nursing team felt defeated and several nurses and nursing technicians were "emotionally burnt out" (quoted from the nursing notes).

The nursing staff organized a special patient care conference, with the psychiatrist as moderator. The staff discussed the strain they felt in caring for the patient and agreed that Mrs. G. would henceforth be assigned a different nurse each day to share the burden. The patient would not be permitted to "fire" nurses she didn't like. If she said she didn't want to have a particular nurse, the nurse was to tell her, "I'm sorry you feel that way, but I will be your nurse today. You'll have a different nurse tomorrow."

Dressing changes were to be done the same way by all nurses. They would be wet to dry, completed in 20 minutes, and the same dose of morphine would be given by each nurse prior to changes. The patient would not be permitted to "help" with the changes. A weekly care conference was organized to discuss her care.

The surgical resident and the nursing supervisor told Mrs. G. that she could cry and curse during dressing changes but that screaming bloody murder disturbed the other patients. They also insisted that she be covered. Round the clock (routine) narcotics were tapered but narcotic analgesics were permitted before dressing changes.

Unfortunately, by the time the psychiatric consultation was ordered, several excellent nurses had come to view each other with distrust and all the consultant could think to do was to invite two of them out for a drink. A fine kettle of fish. Staff splitting might have been avoided had the nurses caring for Mrs. G. held a special staff conference early in the course of her hospitalization to discuss her behavior and their response to it. A significant divergence of opinions about a patient may seriously undermine effective limit setting.

Are we perhaps too cold and hard in our discussion of limit setting? Perhaps you're thinking that, after all, some people simply need more than others and it may be our unwillingness to go the extra mile that leads to all the difficulty in the first place. In reading the next case, think about where you might have set limits. Were we being cruel?

> Ms. A., a tall, attractive redheaded attorney, was admitted to the hospital with a thoracic vertebral fracture and osteomyelitis. She was estranged from her husband and two daughters, in part because they had refused her requests to change their clothing whenever they entered her apartment. She said she was extremely sensitive to chemicals in the environment and demanded a private hospital room, banning the use of all disinfectants and cleaning sprays in the room, insisting on using her own sheets, and requesting special meals and bottled spring water. (She had twenty bottles of spring water in her room at the time of discharge.)
>
> She called the dietary service daily, sometimes three times a day, for meals to be specially prepared but was often unavailable when the food service technician made rounds. Yet she wanted the meal served at her convenience. She might, for example, sleep until 10 am, then request a special breakfast and a special late lunch. The times changed daily.
>
> Her medication had to be given in the precise manner she dictated and she often refused medications.
>
> As she prohibited any cleaning of her room, it became dirty and extremely cluttered. Although she was up and about for the three weeks prior to her discharge, and remained vocal lest staff carelessly contaminate her or her belongings, the mess in her room became odious – 20 pairs of blood-stained underwear in her closet, bits of paper everywhere.
>
> She once reported feeling miserable for 24 hours after Betadine skin cleansing for intravenous line placement, yet the IV report sheet listed Betadine as an allergy

and none was reportedly used, nor were problems or complaints reported during this 24-hour period.

Because of her spinal fracture she wore a brace, the placement of which, normally taking 10 minutes or so, took 45 minutes with her because she insisted that it be positioned perfectly. When she felt rushed she screamed, insisting the entire procedure start from the beginning. She was particularly perfectionistic with new nurses and nursing technicians.

She insisted that, because of pain, she could not attend unassisted to hygiene, toileting, etc. She moved at a snail's pace, stopping at length to talk, so that getting her to the bathroom could take 1 to 2 hours. As the night shift had only four nurses and one technician the patient was asked to use the bedside commode, but she soon refused.

Early in the course of her hospitalization the patient "fired" a nurse who had begun to set limits.

A special assistant was assigned to help her to obtain Medicaid coverage. This young woman came many times but Ms. A. regularly sent her away to ". . . come another time."

As her discharge approached and the names of possible nursing homes were mentioned she called them, interrogating the admitting nurse about the home's ability to meet a long list of her needs, resulting in the screening nurse deciding against accepting the patient.

It became difficult to find people willing to care for her as the demands she made on their time were enormous though her medical condition did not warrant it.

For years she sought no care for vaginal bleeding. When a biopsy this admission revealed endometrial cancer she refused to consent to hysterectomy until faced with discharge. She then called the gynecologist, insisting surgery be performed immediately.

She had many concerns about surgery. The preoperative visits by three different anesthesiologists only increased her questions and requests for more consultation. She asked them to call her ex-husband and explain their techniques to him.

The gynecologist had told her he needed two weeks notice to schedule surgery, but after six weeks of intravenous antibiotic treatment had been completed she had still not consented to a hysterectomy in time to have it scheduled. Ms. A. refused to help in discharge planning and, having made no attempt to complete her application forms for Medicaid, had no insurance coverage for a nursing home stay. Finally, the nursing staff had a conference and set a discharge date. Ms. A. was given 1 week's notice of the discharge date.

She began to work closely with the social worker to find a nursing home. She spoke with the physical and occupational therapists to obtain devices, felt unnecessary by the nursing staff, that would assist her in toileting. Miraculously, or so it seemed, she got her Medicaid application approved by personally making phone calls to the appropriate people to expedite the process.

After the staff meeting, the nurses uniformly became firm about the time needed for applying the brace and the time they had available to spend in the room.

On the day of discharge, though Ms. A.'s nurse told her that the cabulance would arrive to pick her up at 15:45, she made no attempt to pack her things or organize her room and, one hour before discharge, she announced that she could not leave as the technician was to come and adjust her brace. Having spoken with him two days previously, her nurse knew this was untrue, told the patient so, and insisted on discharge as planned.

For six weeks she had refused to change the sheets on her bed and was offended if anyone sat on her bed, lest they "contaminate" the sheets. Then at discharge, as the sheets were being removed from the bed, she became dramatically emotional because they were being improperly folded. She planned to use them in the nursing home unwashed.

Ms. A. would not pack her own belongings, but as the staff began to do so became upset because they were being "contaminated." The staff ignored her. Eventually 12 huge plastic bags were packed.

Anticipating that Ms. A. might put up some last minute barriers to discharge, her nurse called security to accompany the patient from the floor. Until security arrived, Ms. A. would not get off the telephone. As her valuables were collected from the safe downstairs, she accused the hospital of having stolen her checkbook during the admission process. As she was escorted to the cabulance by the driver, the nurse, the transporter, and security, she spoke angrily of having been humiliated by the presence of the security staff since there was no need for it.

At the cabulance, she requested to sit in the front with the driver. Request denied.

A nursing staff conference was held prior to Ms. A.'s readmission for hysterectomy. A letter was composed and sent to the patient. It acknowledged the patient's suffering and expressed the staff's sympathy for her. It then outlined a nursing care plan including mandatory requirements for postoperative care and personal hygiene. The firing of nurses would be disallowed.

During the second admission Ms. A. used hospital sheets without adverse reactions, got up the day after surgery, made many fewer demands. Twice she asked nurses, "Do you think I'm hard to get along with?" She was discharged on time without problems. Nursing management and patient behavior during the second admission were vastly better.

The nurse who largely managed the care of this patient towards the end of her stay was experienced, self-confident, and compassionate but constantly vigilant for patient resistance, dissimulation, and emotional outbursts. Nevertheless, this nurse's perseverance helped the patient, the hospital, and her nursing colleagues. She did it because it was a part, albeit an unpleasant part, of good nursing care. Her colleagues supported her, as did the attending internist.

Agreements or patient care contracts

The patient described in the previous case received a letter outlining expectations. She was expected to comply with requests but was not asked formally to agree.

Sometimes it is necessary formally to ask a patient to agree to conform to expectations.[1] A patient care contract, or agreement is used. Ideally, a physician and ward nurse[2] meet with the patient and draw the contract up in the room. Sometimes, to save time, staff members write the contract before the meeting. We present here an example of an agreement with explicitly stated expectations of behavior and compliance. Each agreement will, of course, be different.

Agreement

The staff here at *City Hospital* wishes to provide you with the best possible care but we are unable to do so unless you do your part to help. Please show us that you accept your responsibilities as a patient by reading and signing this agreement.

I, *patient's name*, understand that I am entitled to the best medical care *City Hospital* can offer. I am entitled to respectful treatment, attention to my comfort, and an explanation of why tests and examinations are ordered. I also understand that I must do my part as a patient and therefore I agree to the following:

I agree not to slam doors when I am angry. (*behavior*)

I agree not to yell at staff members, other patients, or visitors. (*behavior*)

I agree not to threaten staff members, other patients, or visitors. (*behavior*)

I agree to let the staff care for me by taking my blood pressure, pulse, and temperature; by changing my dressings, drawing blood, getting X-rays, and so forth. (*compliance*)

I agree not to smoke in my room. (*compliance*)

I agree not to take any drug, herb, medication, or illicit substance while a patient here unless it is prescribed by one of the hospital doctors. (*compliance*)

I agree to follow the instructions of my nurse or physician. (*compliance*)

I understand that if I do not follow the specifics of this agreement that I may be discharged from the hospital.[3] (*compliance*)

Signed

(Patient's name) . . . .

Date . . . .

Witnessed by . . . .

The tone makes the music as we've noted before, so the staff members presenting this agreement to the patient speak calmly and spend enough time to answer questions.

One must not tell the patient that he will be discharged for breaking the agreement if the physician of record cannot in good conscience actually discharge the patient. Various obstacles may prevent a patient from being discharged, even for obnoxious behavior and non-compliance. A physician may simply be unable to set this sort of limit, or may feel that immediate harm would befall the patient on discharge, or that medical ethics prohibits discharge at this time. The nurse may need to ask the physician what exactly hinders the discharge of an abusive, non-compliant patient.

What then would be the consequences of non-compliance? Perhaps the patient along with reasonable and concerned family members would be informed that the patient will not be accepted in the future for treatment at *City Hospital*.

Disagreement among nurses about whether to set limits

Psychiatric nurses agree that limit setting is important, but in one study by question-naire, at least, experienced nurses were more likely than inexperienced nurses to first choose less restrictive methods to manage conflict before moving to limit setting (Lowe *et al*. 2003). Clearly nurses must respect patient autonomy as much as possible, take an empathic stance, remain calm, allow patients time to reestablish self-control, offer realistic options, and maintain honesty (Lowe 1992). An empathic stance may reduce violence (Lancee *et al*. 1995). As we have mentioned elsewhere, the tone makes the music.

Nurses may have genuine disagreement about the correct approach (Holzworth and Wills 1999) and experienced nurses may be more skilled at defusing dangerous situations. As Lowe and colleagues (2003) note, limit setting occurs in the context of helping patients regain control over themselves without limits, if this is possible. Listening and limit setting go together (DeLaune 1991).

Enforcing limits

In most cases, the nurse enforces the limits simply by being firm, not giving in, enlisting in the struggle his or her nursing colleagues, physicians, and other staff. Remaining firm against a patient's pressure to do otherwise can be difficult but isn't always. Most patients will eventually comply, especially when the staff speaks as one.

There are, sadly, patients who are unwilling or unable to comply with directions. If a patient is so agitated or violent that he poses a threat to himself, to you, or to your staff, then he must be restrained. Often a vest restraint is used for the elderly confused. Sometimes wrist restraints are necessary. You may need several people, even the security staff to help apply them. Each hospital has its own requirements for documentation of necessity.

Restraints need not be limited to the delirious patient. Any patient so obstreperous as to pose a danger may need physical restraints. A borderline patient threatening harm to self or others – and that includes threats to pull out IV lines or to punch the technician – can be told that unless he calms down restraints will be applied to protect him and others. This is not meant to be a threat, just an explanation of consequences of behavior. Document your reasons in the chart in concrete language. Quote the patient if necessary.

We have discussed the use of chemical restraints in various places throughout this book. Intravenous or intramuscular haloperidol or lorazepam may be used. (Note that IM diazepam is poorly absorbed.) A physician will write the orders, but the nurse is most likely the person who will bring the problem to the physician's attention.

Sometimes a show of force is necessary. The hospital security staff along with five to ten strong staff members may need to show themselves so the patient understands there are resources and resolve to do what needs doing, for example, applying restraints, administering medication, or both. Even a small community hospital will have some persons with imposing physique on its staff, with a little luck, even a body builder. These persons should receive some training in techniques for safely restraining a patient.

You may need to enlist family for limit setting. Explain to the family what the patient is doing or saying. "Ms. Forearm is throwing bottles at the nurses" will be viewed by the family as less derogatory than, "Ms. Forearm is really getting mean and dangerous" – not to mention "frustrating, annoying, abusive, bad, or hellish." Ask them to speak with the patient, maybe even spend the night. Let common sense be your guide here.

Seriously ill, medically unstable patients present the biggest challenge to nursing staff wishing to enforce limits. What do you do if all attempts at limit setting fail, and the patient continues to abuse the staff? What if this particular patient, like Ms. Smith, abuses the staff every single time she is admitted to the hospital?

A young woman with diabetes screamed at staff intermittently throughout each hospital stay when her wishes were denied, sometimes using racial epithets or expletives, periodically throwing things, leaving the floor even when expressly told not to, eating sweets in the cafeteria, smoking marijuana in her room, and in general behaving in such a fashion that the nursing staff disliked caring for her but did so, first, because it was their professional duty, and also because she was a patient in need, a poor soul, with, believe it or not, endearing qualities as well as infuriating ones. On admission, she usually was quite ill with ketoacidosis. Her physician was dedicated. Note, however, that he did not have to care for her all shift long.

Various limit setting trials failed, including one attempt to have the patient involuntarily treated in a psychiatric hospital on the basis that she might be a danger to herself or others. During a formal psychiatric evaluation for involuntary commitment she cooly denied suicidality or the wish to harm others.

Hospital stay after hospital stay, her behavior fluctuated – sometimes bad, sometimes very bad. The staff cared for this patient for years until one day she told a nurse that she wouldn't be content until she stabbed the IV technician who, as she put it, had given her a hard time. This time the room was searched and an impressively large, military-style knife was discovered and confiscated.

An experienced staff nurse, who had personally cared about and cared for the patient for years, handling the abuse with aplomb until now, explained to the patient's physician that the staff could no longer care for her. The chief hospital administrator wrote the patient a letter. Care would no longer be provided by this facility.

When patients resist it, setting limits can be hard, emotionally draining work. It is best done as a member of a group with group understanding and group support. Though it is quite hard for those nurses made anxious by confrontation, limit setting is a necessary part of every nurse's work. Practice helps as does self-assurance, but self-assurance comes only with practice.

Knowing the right words to use can be helpful. Avoid language that the patient may misinterpret as blaming. For example, rather than saying, "You shouldn't do that," you might consider saying, "I'm uncomfortable with your doing that." or "You deserve the best care and I'm going to try and provide it."

Don't forget the doctor when it comes to limit setting. It is more effective if you and the doctor have a plan that can be presented jointly to the patient. Not only does it carry more weight coming from both of you, but you will have heard exactly what the doctor said and how the patient responded. The doctor should always be told of inappropriate behavior patterns. When possible, opioid analgesics should be given on a routine rather than a prn schedule, as we never tire of repeating.

Remember limit setting is not scolding, punishing, or belittling the patient. It should be done in a respectful tone. Postponement of appropriate limit setting only makes things worse (Table 10).

Table 10 Limit setting

- Identify the problematic behavior(s)
- Discuss the problem with your colleagues
- Achieve consensus about which behavior should be discouraged and which alternative behavior should be encouraged
- Discuss with the patient what is desirable behavior
- Discuss consequences of desirable and undesirable behavior
- Use a gentle, non-punitive tone and language that is easily understood
- Do not argue or bargain with the patient
- Monitor behavior and institute consequences when appropriate
- Communicate plans, and behavior, to staff day to day and from shift to shift
- (For excessive or inappropriate use of painkillers, tranquilizers, etc., see Chapter 2 on substance abuse.)

Bibliography

Abroms GM. 1968 Setting limits. *Archives of General Psychiatry*. 19(1):113–19, Jul.

Carser D. 1979 The defense mechanism of splitting: developmental origins, effects on staff, recommendations for nursing care. *Journal of Psychiatric Nursing & Mental Health Services*. 17(3):21–8, Mar.

Davidhizar R. 1989 The art of setting limits. *Advancing Clinical Care*. 4(6):26–7, Nov–Dec.

DeLaune SC. 1991 Effective limit setting. How to avoid being manipulated. *Nursing Clinics of North America*. 26(3):757–64, Sep.

Grossman S. 1997 How can nurses use limit setting to facilitate spinal cord patients' independence?. *SCI Nursing*. 14(3):105–7, Sep.

Holzworth RJ. Wills CE. 1999 Nurses' judgments regarding seclusion and restraint of psychiatric patients: a social judgment analysis. *Research in Nursing & Health*. 22(3):189–201, Jun.

Lancee WJ. Gallop R. McCay E. Toner B. 1995 The relationship between nurses' limit-setting styles and anger in psychiatric inpatients. *Psychiatric Services*. 46(6):609–13, Jun.

Levy G. 1993 The art of setting limits. *MEDSURG Nursing*. 2(5):414, 416, Oct.

Lowe T. 1992 Characteristics of effective nursing interventions in the management of challenging behaviour. *Journal of Advanced Nursing.* 17(10):1226–32, Oct.

Lowe T. Wellman N. Taylor R. 2003 Limit-setting and decision-making in the management of aggression. *Journal of Advanced Nursing.* 41(2):154–61, Jan.

Lyon GG. 1970 Limit setting as a therapeutic tool. *Journal of Psychiatric Nursing & Mental Health Services.* 8(6):17–21, Nov–Dec.

Pam A. 1994 Limit setting: theory, techniques, and risks. *American Journal of Psychotherapy.* 48(3):432–40, Summer.

Sharrock J. Rickard N. 2002 Limit setting: a useful strategy in rehabilitation. *Australian Journal of Advanced Nursing.* 19(4):21–6, Jun–Sep.

Zollo MB. Derse A. 1997 The abusive patient: where do you draw the line? *American Journal of Nursing.* 97(2):31–5; quiz 36, Feb.

Chapter 6

The nurse's authority

Nurses play different roles in different settings: caregiver, teacher, patient advocate, administrator, counselor, morale booster, etc. The nurse's effectiveness in each of these roles depends, in part, on both the patient's and the nurse's awareness of the nurse's authority.

"Authority" has several meanings: (1) The *power* to influence or persuade resulting from knowledge or experience; (2) the *power* to enforce laws, exact obedience, command, determine, or judge; (3) an accepted source of *expertise* or advice; and (4) *confidence* derived from experience or practice; firm self-assurance (American Heritage Dictionary).

In this chapter we discuss various facets of the nurse's power (definitions 1 and 2), expertise (3), and confidence (4), though not necessarily in that order.

Professional identity and confidence

Professional identity may be described as the belief that one can practice nursing with skill and responsibility (Fagermoen 1997; Ohlen and Segesten 1998). Caring for patients requires compassion, competence, and confidence (Roach 1992). Confidence and professional identity may be weakened when the unprepared nurse is challenged by the difficult patient.

> Sam Button is on the call light again for the sixteenth time this shift and for the sixteenth time Kathy Sant, R.N., enters the room with a smile on her face, though it has begun to droop. Mr. Button wrecked his car while drunk and now has two broken legs and sundry other injuries. "Could you get me my magazine, honey?" he asks, pointing to the magazine within reach on the table next to his bed. Last visit he asked Ms. Sant to help him place a phone call to "a business associate", and the two or three times before that to complain drowsily that he wasn't getting enough pain killer and that the other nurses didn't know what they were doing, though Ms. Sant herself was "a sweetheart". He wondered aloud, however, what unnecessary preoccupation might be keeping her away so long when he needed her. He is quick to anger.
>
> She gets Mr. Button his magazine and leaves. The call light is on again shortly and she returns, her smile a mere shadow of its former self. "Would you take a look at my belly? It's hurting," he asks. He always has the top of his hospital gown off so he can display his chest, but getting a good look at his abdomen requires

the removal of a complicated dressing. The surgeons were in a while ago. She examined his abdomen earlier in the day. She's about to go off shift so she politely puts him off as he begins to offer a description of the problem. She performs no examination. She forgets to mention his complaint to the nurse coming on duty. The next morning she returns to find that he's gone to the operating room having developed an intra-abdominal hemorrhage.

What feelings are elicited by this vignette? How would your confidence have been affected under similar circumstances? How would such feelings have affected your decision to examine Mr. Button? Might you have blamed the patient? What action on the nurse's part might have made Mr. Button easier to care for?

What happens to the nurse's confidence, when belittled, manipulated, or clung to? How does a nurse feel when a patient questions his or her competence or fails to respond to measures that help other patients? Metaphorical dragons in the hospital have a metaphorical bite that causes real pain.

In J. K. Rowling's *Harry Potter and the Sorcerer's Stone*, Hagrid, the gamekeeper at a school for wizards, is an enormous, gentle man with a penchant for dangerous magical creatures. He decides to raise a baby dragon. Though still small, it is fearsome. Its bite is painful and poisonous, causing wounds that fester, but after it bites Hagrid he continues to care for it with no less dedication than before. This, however, is a children's story.

Wounds to professional identity may make caring for patients like Mr. Button difficult for the nurse and they may linger making future care of similar patients difficult.

The nurse's authority

Qualms about the exercise of authority make caring for recalcitrant patients even more difficult. Some nurses feel that such expression is authoritarian, mean, or niggling. Some feel it is not compassionate, some that it is a sign of their failure with the patient. Yet until the nurse can comfortably exercise authority, she or he will be ineffective with difficult patients. Intellectual acceptance of one's authority is only a start. Exercising authority must feel right. It must be exercised again and again, until the benefits are clear and the nurse is comfortable with it. Nurses should use benevolent power (Fisher and Davidhizar 1998; Davidhizar and Dowd 1999).

We do not advocate authoritarianism, the demand for unquestioning obedience, the abrogation of individual freedom. On the contrary, we, like you, know that both nursing and medical care are poorer without the patient's active participation. Nevertheless, the nurse is a licensed professional, an officially acknowledged source of information about the patient's illness and treatment; she has the responsibility to influence the patient and the power to enforce the rules – and with time should develop self-assurance in these matters. With most patients the question of authority is never raised. The average patient is grateful and cooperative, understanding and accepting of the nurse's authority.

Most nurses go into the profession for the satisfaction that the knowledge, skills, and caring provide. Exercising their authority with recalcitrant patients was never their goal. But if these patients are going to get the best nursing care possible, as they themselves wish, they will need to comply with the care plan that is in their best interests.

Authority does not imply cruelty, an angry tone of voice, disregard for the rights of others, or other sundry undesirable behaviors. With a voice like an angel, one can confront a patient smoking in the bathroom, not to mention shooting up under the blankets.

You are less likely to be flustered by an obstreperous patient if you are self-confident. You words, tone of voice, and actions will be self-assured. Unfortunately this self-confidence derives principally from experience. We say "unfortunately" because experience takes time and involves making mistakes, referred to by some as the school of hard knocks. Still, your distress at mistakes may lead to better retention of the lessons learned by making them. Only by having managed a sufficient number of patients with sufficiently diverse problems will you come to feel that, in most cases, you really know what you are doing.

Perhaps if Nurse Sant had exerted her authority early on in the care of Mr. Button by setting limits on his language and demands, she would have been less frustrated with him and more likely to note a real change in his clinical condition. A key part of this book is about setting limits, but in order to do so effectively a nurse must have some confidence in doing so.

Humor

Our tone of voice affects how our message is received. Put another way, the tone makes the music. Authority shouldn't be exercised by growling. If, for example, a father with mock sadness and a hitch in his voice, sniffling a bit, tells his teenage son to "Please do the dishes," his son is less likely to bite his head off than if he snarls out an order. The boy may respond to such underspoken irony not only by remaining calm but by actually doing the dishes.

The successful parent, in this case, has exercised his authority – he has asked his son to do the dishes – without eliciting either reflex resistance or acute catatonia. Such an approach has little risk. If it fails, for example, the parent's mock sadness may quickly deteriorate into genuine blubbering, at which point many sons turn automatically to do the dishes.

The ironic stance, used cautiously, may not only amuse the potential dishwasher but the potentially non-compliant patient as well. The nurse may wipe her eyes with a handkerchief, beseeching the patient to save specimens of his sputum, or emesis, or urine lest she have a nervous breakdown. Alternatively, the nurse might say, "It must be very precious to you. You won't give us any." One must find one's own style.

Nursing literature is replete with articles on the use of humor to relax the anxious patient, establish rapport, enhance teaching, or provide relief (see James 1995).

Perhaps the simplest way to introduce humor into your practice is to learn a few jokes or amusing stories by heart. For success, keep three things in mind:

- First, your timing should be right. Is the patient ready for a joke? Are there distractions? Is the patient in too much distress?
- Second, the patient must be receptive. You may ask, "Do you like jokes or funny stories?" " Do you laugh out loud or just smile at jokes?"
- Third, your stories should be appropriate. Don't make jokes about the patient. Don't tell jokes which ridicule a particular race, ethnicity, religion, or sex. For example:

"How do you make holy water?" You boil the hell out of it." (Is this joke a violation of our own rules?)

"Why do seagulls fly over the sea and not the bay? Because then they'd be bagels."

An old woman at the airline: "I'm going to Los Angeles. I'd like you to send this bag to Chicago and this one to New York."

The agent says, "Madam, we can't do that."

"Why not, you did it last trip."

"Did you hear the one about the farmer's daughter . . ."

No. Don't tell this joke (Dowd *et al*. 2003) (see Table 11, boundary violations).

Anyone can employ humor to relax, distract, engage, or parry the difficult patient, but we can offer no more than a few examples. You can tell jokes to your colleagues, too. They are a form of exchange and if you tell a joke you are likely to be told one in return.

Humor rarely has a place if you are verbally or physically attacked by an angry patient. Then either focused listening or limit setting is in order. When the smoke has cleared, however, humor might have a role in reestablishing a relationship. Humor is most likely to help in the context of a trusting relationship between nurse and patient. The use of humor does not diminish authority.

Professional distance (also referred to as professional boundaries)

A good nurse cares about the patient as a person. An uncaring nurse is, at best, an efficient technician. He is unable to care for the whole person. The good nurse, in the course of his duties, learns something of the patient's interests, values, talents, and so on. Meeting the family, hearing stories about the patient, and making small talk all play a role. The nurse expresses the appropriate amount of compassion and concern.

It does not follow, however, that the more the nurse cares about the patient, the better and better the care becomes. We can't describe the threshold, but with emotional over-attachment a nurse's judgment and effectiveness begin to falter. The extreme is easy to illustrate. How good would you be at administering chemotherapy to your own resistant child, spouse, or partner or weaning them from narcotics on which they had become dependent?

When we speak of professional distance we do not mean aloofness, emotional detachment, cold objectivity. We mean the right distance: caring enough about the person that his well-being remains foremost in your mind, but not so much that your objectivity is impaired. Professional distance, then, means the optimal amount of emotional involvement to provide good care. This distance may be difficult or impossible to measure and it varies from nurse to nurse.

Too great a distance also impairs objectivity, because the patient is no longer valued as a person. If you truly cannot abide a particular patient, be honest with yourself and consider finding a colleague to care for them. (Because there are persons you cannot tolerate says little about you. As the perversion of an old song title goes – "Everybody hates somebody sometime.")

There are patients that neither you, nor any of your colleagues, can long abide, and sometimes it is necessary to share among yourselves the burden of caring for such poor souls. Although assigning the same nurse each day to care for the difficult patient is usually recommended, and we do recommend it, rotating assignments may occasionally be necessary for the well-being of the staff. Rotating caregivers should be a last resort, however.

"Professional boundaries" is a term very closely related to the concept of "professional distance", but more often used to discuss inappropriate closeness rather than inappropriate distance (Smith *et al.* 1997). Because some difficult patients, especially those with personality disorders, themselves may tend to develop inappropriate feelings toward their nurse, that is, tend to cross the boundary between being a patient and being a friend of the nurse, nurses must be aware of their own feelings. The National Council of State Boards of Nursing, Inc., outlines how a nurse can identify potential boundary violations and we include here a table from that pamphlet (Table 11).

Table 11 Potential boundary violations[a]

- Inappropriate self-disclosure – the nurse discusses intimate thoughts and feelings with the patient
- Secretive behavior – the nurse keeps secrets with patient or is guarded about their interactions
- "Super nurse" behavior – the nurse believes that only he or she understands and meets the patient's needs and that nothing between them could ever be non-therapeutic
- Special patient treatment or patient attention to the nurse – the nurse spends inappropriate lengths of time with the patient, visits when off duty, trades assignments to be with the patient. Or the patient pays special attention to the nurse, e.g., buying gifts
- Selective communications – the nurse fails to explain aspects of care or reports only some aspects of the patient's behavior or the patient returns repeatedly to the nurse because other staff members are "too busy"
- Flirtations – the nurse communicates in a flirtatious manner, perhaps employing sexual innuendo or off-color jokes
- "You and me against the world" behavior – the nurse is overly protective of the patient and sides with him or her regardless of the situation
- Failure to protect patient – the nurse fails to recognize feelings of sexual attraction to the patient, consult with a colleague or supervisor, or transfer care of the patient to support boundary integrity

Source: National Council of State Boards of Nursing, Inc. 1996.

Note
[a] We have used the word "patient" in this table rather than "client" as was used in the original publication.

As that pamphlet notes, "boundary violations are extremely complex". We are unable to discuss them in detail here.

Staff meetings, staff plans, staff interventions

The nurse's authority – power, expertise, and confidence – is strengthened by strong bonds and good communication with the other nurses on the staff. Clearly if one nurse tries single-handedly to change the problematic behavior of a patient, failure is more likely than if a united staff – day, evening, and night shifts – work together with the same plan of action. Although staff meetings are more likely to occur at shift change from day to evening, the night shift staff will hear about the day's events from the evening staff at the next change of shift.

A nurse confronted with a difficult patient may assume that the problem is between the two of them and hence keep her distress to herself. We believe, however, that *even a flicker of recognition of difficulty* should lead the nurse to raise the question with a trusted colleague, or better still, at a staff meeting or case conference. This may be difficult because the nurse may have only a vague feeling of unease about the patient, unable to put her finger on the problem. One may say, "I don't know what it is, but I have a funny feeling caring for Mr. Mellacreesent. How about you?"

If several people openly call Mr. Mellacreesent difficult or manipulative, the subject should be raised at a meeting. Leslie Nield-Andersen, Ph.D., APRN, and colleagues, in an article on manipulative, sexually provocative, and aggressive patients provide numerous practical suggestions for care plans and note that when the staff doesn't address undesirable patient behaviors together, the behaviors continue (Nield-Anderson *et al.* 1999).

Nurses at the meeting may begin by offering concrete examples of how the patient behaves with them, their reactions, and the patient's responses. Making a care plan for difficult patients is easiest, of course, when everyone identifies the same behaviors as problematic and when their cause, even if not perfectly clear, is generally understood.

Then a standard approach can be outlined in the nursing care plan and the staff can monitor the patient's response.

Inconsistency feeds a fire: if one nurse calls the doctor whenever the patient asks but another does not; if one nurse gives prn uptidduptine or snoozerooziam whenever the patient asks, but another does not; if one nurse allows the patient to go out to smoke whenever the patient asks but another does not; if one nurse excuses the patient from PT but another does not; if one nurse tolerates sexual innuendo but another does not; and so ad infinitum. As a team you may decide to leave some things fully to the nurse's discretion, to set limits on others, to forbid some things outright.

Sometimes it just helps if every nurse uses the same words in explaining limits. If, for example, the team decides that the doctor should not be called every time the patient asks, you might all agree on the wording for refusing the request, "Mr. Mellacreesent, I'm uncomfortable calling the doctor for this right now because I believe your condition is stable but I'll be sure he learns about this as soon as possible." For sexually tinged small talk or flirting, "Mr. Mellacreesent, it makes me uncomfortable when you talk about '(fill in the blank)'. Please don't."

Although you may be able to set objective parameters on when to give a prn medication, you might consider having prn's eliminated altogether and replaced with routinely administered medication. We address the question of prn uptidduptine and snoozerooziam in Chapter 2 on substance abuse.

Although it may appear unnecessary to invite the attending physician or managing medical or surgical resident to the meeting, it's best that he or she hears what the nursing staff is facing. The moderating nurse begins by stating how long the meeting will last, concisely describing the reason for the meeting, then asking the physician to briefly outline the pertinent medical facts and the plan. That may be all that's needed of the physician so she may be excused if necessary. This is, however, an opportunity for the staff to ask the physician questions that will aid them in their management of the patient. They may wish to know how much pain would ordinarily be experienced from such and such a dressing change, or how precarious the patient's respiratory drive really is, or how one should understand a complaint that is far out of proportion to what would be expected.

The nurse who is confused about a patient's medical condition will be insecure with any patient, but especially with the challenging patients we are talking about. That's why the physician should present the case at the start of the meeting.

If it appears that a behavioral contract and strict limit setting will be needed to get the patient's behavior under control, the doctor should be asked if she would be comfortable discharging the patient should attempts at behavioral control fail.[1]

Today the management of a patient's admission, treatment, and discharge from the hospital is more complicated than ever before. Nurses, physicians, pharmacists, dieticians, physical and occupational therapists, respiratory therapists, and medical social workers are all necessary. The medical social worker is often key for smooth discharge and should always be included in such meetings. Each of these members has something to contribute. Remember that your job may be easier if the physical therapist's job is and vice versa.

When a meeting is necessary, one nurse should be responsible for making a list of attendees, outlining the problem, and moderating the meeting, and asking someone to take notes and summarize the new nursing plan. She may wish, however, to delegate to the health unit coordinator or ward clerk the task of calling the potential attendees.

Remember it's probably better to have a meeting than not to, even if not everyone can attend. One person should have the responsibility of organizing the meeting, but you may wish to rotate the responsibility.

In some cases nurses may be surprised to discover that the patient is charming with some of them, and insufferable with others. Such a gross disparity in behaviors often indicates that the patient is idealizing some nurses and devaluing others, and that the idealized and devalued nurses, the "good" and the "bad" nurses, are responding to the patient accordingly. This is called staff splitting. It's bad news.

Not everyone on the staff necessarily likes everyone else (Taylor 2001). We all have our rivalries, our vanities, our likes and our dislikes. And, of course, some nurses are better than others with some patients. Nevertheless, nurses must be on guard not to assume that their colleague is just no good with Mr. Mellacreesent or, the shoe on the other foot, that their colleague only gets along with Mr. Mellacreesent because she panders to him. Of course, the better you know and respect your colleagues, and the more group cohesion there is on your unit, the less likely are these suspicions and resentments.

If most staff members call for limit setting, the "good" nurse may worry that the staff is being punitive or uncaring. Even if the staff agrees that Mr. Mellacreesent's behavior has split the staff, the "good" nurse may continue to feel positively toward him and may have some difficulty setting the agreed upon limits, whereas the "bad" nurse may continue to harbor some resentment. Continued discussion may help resolve discordant feelings. Achieving the right professional distance from the onset is also protective. It should be perfectly clear by our use of quotation marks that neither nurse can be judged good or bad based on how she is perceived by a certain patient.

It is important that the staff come to a real consensus about what nurses should and should not do and say in working with the patient. Each nurse should approach the patient in basically the same way, with the same expectations, the same limits, the same willingness to confront the patient with unacceptable behaviors. Consistency is paramount. The patient's behavior will not improve if some nurses adhere to the limits while others don't. The less cohesive the nurses on a floor, the more easily are the seeds of discord sewn among them. Though it may sound melodramatic – hostility, power struggles, and conflict ensue if consensus cannot be reached about patient management. This is another sign of splitting. Diplomacy is needed in discussing these matters so that nurses will not feel they are being labeled.

If you are the only one out of sync with your colleagues, consider counter-transference.[2]

Talking with your colleagues about patient care is important for obvious reasons: meetings teach you about nursing in general, and about nursing care in particular cases. Such meetings also help establish your identity and authority as a nurse. We need not belabor these points here. Periodically through this book we mention in relation to specific cases, that a staff meeting was held. Such meetings are particularly important in the management of difficult patients.

Nurse–physician communication

A doctor died and went to heaven. Standing at the back of a long line leading to the pearly gates he quickly became impatient. When St. Peter came by, the doctor cornered him and said, "Say, I'm a doctor. Can't I just go to the head of the line?"

"No," said St. Peter, "You'll have to wait your turn like everyone else." Just then the doctor saw someone in a white coat up ahead, with a stethoscope in the pocket, cut in front of the line and walk through the gates. "Hey, that doctor just cut in!", he protested. St. Peter glanced over and then said, "That wasn't a doctor. That was God. He just thinks He's a doctor."

This is an old joke and as Bob Dylan once sang, "the times they are a-changin'". Many physicians are now women and more men are entering nursing. (We defer to theologians the question of God's gender.) Furthermore, younger generations of physicians are less likely than their older colleagues to project god-like superiority. Relatively few physicians are dismissive nowadays, but some are difficult to engage because they are too busy. As a nurse, however, you must still engage them. Decide what you need, put it into words in your own mind, have available the data the doctor may ask for, and then act.

> "Dr. Avatar, I'd like to speak with you for a moment about Mr. Beelzey in room 666. It would really help me and the other nurses if you would. . . ."
> "If I would what?"
> ". . . if you would tell Mr. Beelzey that I am responsible for his nursing care and that you'd appreciate it if he'd cooperate with me."
> ". . . if you would discontinue prn orders for morphine."
> ". . . if you would write for routinely scheduled analgesics."
> ". . . if you would invite me in when you talk to Mr. Beelzey so I can hear the plan and how he responds."

"... if you would explain the plan to me."

"... if you would tell Mr. Beelzey that he must get out of bed once a day."

"... if you would order some IV haloperidol orders for Mr. Beelzey."

"... if you would tell Mr. Beelzey that you wish to be called only if I think it is clinically necessary."

"... if you would tell Mr. Beelzey that you want him to take his medication."

"... if you would explain to Mr. Beelzey that you've worked with me for 16 years and that you trust me, damn it."

Nursing for all patients, not just difficult patients, is much easier and more satisfying when the nurse has the backing of the physician (see Chapter 10, Communicating with doctors).

Bibliography

American Heritage Dictionary. 3rd Edn. 1992. Boston: Houghton Mifflin Co.

Davidhizar R. Dowd SB. 1999 Benevolent power. *Journal of Practical Nursing.* 49(1):24–30; quiz 31–3, Mar.

Davidhizar R. Lonser G. 2003 A carefully delivered introduction. Enhancing style through a carefully delivered introduction. *Journal of Practical Nursing.* 53(4):17–20, Winter.

Davidhizar R. Shearer R. 1998 Improving your bedside manner. *Journal of Practical Nursing.* 48(1):10–14, Mar.

Dowd S. Davidhizar R. Davidhizar R. 2003 Sexuality, sexual harassment, and sexual humor: guidelines for the workplace in health care. *Health Care Manager.* 22(2):144–51, Apr–Jun.

Fagermoen MS. 1997 Professional identity: values embedded in meaningful nursing practice. *Journal of Advanced Nursing.* 25(3):434–41, Mar.

Fisher L. Davidhizar R. 1998 Every nurse is a leader. *Journal of Practical Nursing.* 48(2):16–19, Jun.

James DH. 1995 Humor: a holistic nursing intervention. *Journal of Holistic Nursing.* 13(3), 239–47.

National Council of State Boards of Nursing, Inc., 1996 *Professional Boundaries. A nurse's guide to the importance of appropriate professional boundaries.* 676 N. St. Clair St., Suite 550, Chicago, Ill. 60611–2921.

Nield-Anderson L. Minarik PA. Dilworth JM. Jones J. Nash PK. O'Donnell KL. Steinmiller EA. 1999 Responding to 'difficult' patients. *American Journal of Nursing.* 99(12):26–34.

Ohlen J. Segesten K. 1998 The professional identity of the nurse: concept analysis and development. *Journal of Advance Nursing* 28(4):720–7.

Roach SMS. 1992 *The Human Act of Caring. A Blueprint for the Health Profession.* Ottawa: Canadian Hospital Association Press.

Smith LL. Taylor BB. Keys AT. Gornto SB. 1997 Nurse–patient boundaries: crossing the line. *American Journal of Nursing.* 97(12):26–31; quiz 32, Dec.

Taylor B. 2001 Identifying and transforming dysfunctional nurse–nurse relationships through reflective practice and action research. *International Journal of Nursing Practice.* 7(6):406–13, Dec.

Chapter 7

Manipulation, clinging, sexual provocation, anger, and violence – the feelings they evoke and the interventions they may require

To provide good care for our patients we must be aware of our feelings towards them. The greater our awareness, the less likely we are to allow our feelings to interfere with the quality of our care. When we provide good care despite troubling emotions, difficult patients become less so, and may cease being difficult altogether.

Clinging, demanding, rejecting, denying

Feeling good about the care we provide, however, usually means knowing that it is good, or appreciated care, or effective care. Providing good, effective care to patients who cling, demand, or reject care is difficult but feasible. The nurse's emotional response to such patients depends on their behavior. Underlying many of these behaviors is insatiable dependence as described in "Taking care of the hateful patient" (Groves 1978).

> Anna, a 19-year-old girl with diabetes out of control, is pleasant, sweet, and grateful – excessively grateful. She has many questions about the care she is receiving, and makes it difficult to leave the room. The nurses caring for her feel she's sticky, needy. She calls frequently, as did Sam Button, for reassurance, position changes, to ask questions.

Anna's clinging *may* evoke in the nurse the wish to avoid her. It may be enough to set limits on her expectations.

> Strom Ostermiener, a 56-year-old construction foreman, status post-lung resection for cancer, expects an immediate response when he expresses his wish to see his doctor, his nurse, his physical therapist or to have his morphine, his coffee, his newspaper. He feels entitled to have all his wishes met and all met promptly. He has been angry with the nursing staff and medical staff.

Because he *demands* care, he may evoke in the nurse a wish to attack him. "Who do you think you are anyway, King Tut?" Rather than challenging his sense of entitlement it may be more effective to redirect it. "I know you've been through a lot and have a right to be mad. You're entitled to the best nursing care and we're trying to provide it. We want you to get well but using all that energy to fight us isn't the best thing for your recovery. And it makes it harder caring for you, too."

Another category of "hateful" patient, is the help rejecter, the patient who cannot be satisfied no matter what you do, but whose condition is relatively benign and whose complaints are far out of proportion to what is expected. These patients may evoke depression in their caregivers. Try telling them that it is indeed unlikely that lasting comfort can be obtained but that you're going to try anyway.

Consider also the alcohol dependent patient, admitted repeatedly for bleeding gastric varices, receiving gallons of blood products each visit, but returning to drinking after each discharge. The self-destructive patient in denial may trigger in the nurse who has cared for him repeatedly actual malice: "Why doesn't he just die?"

Most of us have little or no control over the feelings we have towards others, but fortunately, not our feelings but rather our competence, actions, intentions, and tone determine whether we provide good care. It is better to know that a patient evokes malice in us, than to not know it. The good nurse, a professional, will not let such feelings interfere with appropriate care.

Manipulation

You may recognize in many of the case histories in this book a frequent, annoying behavior, namely manipulation. Manipulation means to influence or manage deviously. We become irritated when we realize we are being manipulated because we feel we are being toyed with or discounted. Manipulation is in a sense dishonest. Though we may all be guilty of it from time to time, we will spare you a treatise on the moral state of mankind and simply illustrate some manipulative behaviors seen in the general hospital.

To flatter someone is to compliment them excessively and often insincerely in order to win favor. Unfortunately, we are all susceptible to it if the flatterer truly understands us. Who does not appreciate a compliment about something they are proud of? Who will not be more favorably disposed toward the person who has the discernment to recognize our achievement? Later, when the flatterer asks us for a favor we may be more inclined to go along with it, not wishing to disappoint the discerning person who so appreciates our good qualities. With a little experience though, the nurse quickly sees excessive compliments as a red flag, a warning to be careful.

"I've never had such a good nurse before."
(silent thoughts) Right, 27 previous hospitalizations, 68 previous nurses and never one like me before.
Later, "I know the doctor said I should stay here this afternoon, but could I please just go downstairs for a few minutes?"

If you don't recognize flattery for what it is, you may have more trouble setting limits than you should.

If the patient reserves flattery for some nurses, and disdain for others, and if the nurses on the floor communicate poorly among themselves, trouble is brewing. The flattered nurse may feel well disposed towards the patient, especially if the patient is cooperative and pleasant with her, whereas the disdained nurse will feel resentment, especially if the patient is uncooperative and unpleasant with her. This may lead the "good nurse" to think the "bad nurse" is insensitive or inept while leading the "bad nurse" to think the "good nurse" is softheaded. Ugh. Both may be good nurses, no quotation marks needed. Staff conferences on difficult patients can avoid the discord caused by such staff splitting.

Exaggeration of complaints or plain lying is also manipulative. Sometimes they are used to avoid something felt to be onerous, like physical therapy, other times to obtain narcotics or tranquilizers. The nurse must assess the complaint objectively, if possible.

Frequent calls so that the nurse will be in constant attendance may be manipulative.

Constant anger or hostility is manipulative if it fits the definition, i.e., if it is a devious means of managing or influencing others. Perhaps it is meant to keep the nurse out of the room as much as possible or to get faster service or to intimidate the nurse into giving more analgesics. (See Table 12.)

Rejection of offered care may be manipulative

Some patients get angry when they do not receive what they feel entitled to receive and they feel entitled to receive everything they wish to receive, which means, of course, that they get angry whenever they don't get what they wish.

Because most compliments, complaints, and expressions of anger are legitimate, honest expressions, it is often the nurse's gut reaction, speaking colloquially, which indicates if something is amiss or not. We have similarly used the term "red flag". It takes clinical judgment to recognize when behavior is manipulative and when it is not.

Sexually inappropriate behavior

Nield-Anderson (1999) and colleagues list a number of provocative behaviors including flattery, flirting, exposure of genitals, touching, suggestive remarks, sexual jokes, personal inquiries, etc. They list interventions as well, including clarification for the patient of the nurse's role, redirecting the patient, documenting interactions, confrontation, consulting with colleagues, assessing cultural factors, assessing for delirium or substance abuse, encouraging anxiety reduction techniques, and setting limits.

"Please, Mr. Grope, be more careful where you put your hands."

If a patient's speech or actions make you uncomfortable, you will need to find the right words and tone of voice to say so, words and tone that are firm, yet gentle. This is easiest, of course, if a patient is obviously obscene or indecent. Dealing with gross impropriety is relatively straightforward because the problem is evident and it is easier to take early action. Delaying action makes it harder to do so later, in part, because one may then be more concerned about the patient's reaction. The patient may not understand why you didn't say something sooner.

When the problem is subtler and you are unsure of what you are feeling, you should seek out the help of your colleagues.

Anger

Emotions evolved in mammals as a means of communication. It is of survival value for one animal to know how another is feeling – amorous, angry, frightened? Emotions

Table 12 Nursing interventions for manipulative behavior

Manipulative behavior	Examples or definitions
• Staff splitting	• Idealizing some nurses, devaluing others
• Inappropriate criticism of staff	
• Excessive demands	
• Rejection of care	
• Constant complaints about care	
• Threatening of staff	• Frequent calls to administrators, threats to have the nurse fired
• Requesting more help than is needed	
• Lying	
• Instantly assuming intimacy with caregivers	• Inappropriate self-disclosure, inappropriate inquiry into the private life of the nurse
• Flattery	
• Rudeness or exaggerated anger	
Interventions	
• Set limits	• (see Chapter 5 on limit setting)
• Identify, discuss with staff, and document the problematic behaviors	
• Decide on interventions including limits and document them in the care plan. Monitor their effectiveness.	
• Communicate daily with all staff involved in the patient's care	
• Allow patients some control	• "Would you like your bath now or in half an hour?"
• Teach patients to be direct	• "Mr. Loud, please ask me when you need something rather than calling someone else"
• Communicate between shifts so the approach to the patient remains consistent	
• Arrange team conferences to discuss the patient's care	

Source: Modified from Nield-Anderson *et al.* (1999).

communicate themselves directly. Other things being equal, if you're with a person who is calm, you will tend to be calm. If you are with a person who is sad, you will tend to be sad. And if you are with a person who is angry, you will tend to be angry. Well, either angry or frightened, since these two emotions are intimately, and biochemically, related to each other. If you're feeling anger you will have a tendency to discharge it, that is, attack. If you're feeling frightened, you will have a tendency to escape. These tendencies are often called "fight or flight". Neither facilitates good listening.

If your emotional response is tolerable and you are aware of the need to listen, you will hear the person out, and hence allow the person to reduce his own anger by expressing it. The nurse must not only listen to allow the patient to ventilate, and to understand the patient's concern, but also to categorize more broadly the patient's problem and assess the potential for violence.

In broad outline these patients can be divided up into the following categories:

- The patient who has become frightened or upset because of something that happened.
- The chronically angry or easy to anger patient who is otherwise cognitively intact and not a member of the next three groups.
- The delirious, agitated patient (see Chapter 3 on delirium). Although there may be an incident that leads to the anger, fear and anger are inherent in many deliria.
- The intoxicated patient or patient in alcohol or drug withdrawal.
- The patient with a major psychiatric disorder such as bipolar disorder (manic depressive illness), schizophrenia, Alzheimer's disease, antisocial personality disorder, and others.

Knowing which category your patient belongs in helps you find the right strategy to manage the anger. Although listening may still be helpful for patients in the last three categories, the chances of violence may be greater.

A little anger or hostility is something we all encounter in our day-to-day lives.

The Human Resources department of our hospital distributed a mnemonic for recalling what to do when faced with a patient's or colleague's anger: Take the HEAT:

- Hear the person out.
- Empathize with the person's feelings.
- Accept some responsibility.
- Take action to help ameliorate the situation.

Hearing the person out, listening, is often the most effective thing you can do. Prematurely trying to remedy the situation prevents the person from expressing himself. Yet listening is also often the most difficult thing to do since another person's anger roils our own emotions.

A 27-year-old carpenter convinced he had a serious undiagnosed intra-abdominal lesion was incensed at what he considered the dismissive tone of his attending physician. Without raising his voice the patient spoke about having been denied a CT scan of the abdomen. He had just "fired" his doctor, a person the nurse knew to be a good physician. She felt a boiling up in the pit of her stomach and the urge to reprimand the patient, who clearly didn't know what he was talking about, but she knew that her anger was a signal that the patient's anger was much greater than his tone of voice would suggest. She listened to him for about 5 minutes and then, without agreeing with him about what was needed, told him it sounded like a very difficult situation. He told her she was the only one who seemed to know what she was doing around here. His anger was still present but much diminished.

If you understand your own response to anger you can consciously maintain a calm exterior so that you do not inadvertently exacerbate the patient's distress. Remember that just as the patient's emotions will influence yours, so will yours influence the patient's. You should try to remain calm. You must try to look and sound non-threatening. If it is safe to do so, consider sitting down rather than standing over the patient. Use the HEAT mnemonic if appropriate but *when anger seems excessive* you must make an extra effort to reduce the chance of violence.

Violence

Nurses must attend to their feelings lest these feelings interfere with the provision of good care. Another, no less important, reason is that heeding feelings such as fear can protect nurses from injury by potentially violent patients. If you are frightened by a patient, you *must* heed your fear, assess the risk of violence, and communicate your discomfort to the staff. In addition to your emotional response, you should take into account behaviors indicating an increased chance of violence. Remember that the best predictor of future violence is past violence. For this reason, a nurse against whom aggressive behavior or violence is directed must effectively communicate this to the staff both orally and in writing. Slapping, pushing, biting, spitting, not to mention punching, and throwing things, is violence.

Violence may be heralded by aggressive behavior that signals excessive anger or fear including: tense muscles, reddening or blanching of the face, loud speech, heavy breathing, glaring, profanity, insults, threats, pacing, and threatening posture (Nield-Anderson *et al.* 1999).

Verbal de-escalation of the aggressive behavior is outlined in an article by Dr. Avrim Fishkind (2002), the director of a psychiatric hospital in Houston. His rules and illustrations, somewhat modified, are presented in Table 13. The following discussion derives principally from that article.

The term "in your face" describes behavior in which an aggressive person violates the personal space of another. As Meredith Wilson says in *The Music Man*, some people can "stand touching noses for a week at a time and never see eye-to-eye." Most of us dislike being treated like this. The angry patient certainly will. Stay at two arms' length so you won't get hit and so the patient doesn't feel threatened. Neither avert your eyes, which may signal fear to the patient, nor stare at him or her, which may be perceived as aggressive. Leave a clear path for escape which either you or the patient can use.

Remember that just as the patient's emotions and behavior will affect yours, so will yours affect the patient's. You should assume a casual posture, leaving relaxed, open hands at your side or on your lap. Allow your facial muscles to relax so you appear calm even if you don't feel it. Use a calm, gentle tone. Dr. Fishkind suggests imagining yourself with a patient you like and expressing concern as you would with such a patient. Never threaten the patient.

The emotions of anger and fear generally make it very difficult to listen at all, much less to listen dispassionately. They usually lead to fight or flight. Just picture yourself in a setting in which you are angry or frightened. How well would you listen?

In order for the angry person to hear and understand what you are saying you should be concise and repetitive. Agitated patients, especially if delirious or psychotic, will have even more trouble listening.

Table 13 Nine rules for the verbal de-escalation of anger

Rule	Explanation
• Respect personal space	• Stay at two arms' length. Maintain usual social eye contact. (Neither stare nor avert your gaze.) Don't block an escape route for either you or the patient
• Do not provoke the patient	• Maintain a calm demeanor and stance. Speak softly. Do not threaten
• Be concise and repeat yourself	• Use short phrases or sentences. Use a simple vocabulary. Repeat yourself as often as necessary
• Recognize the patient's wants and feelings	• "You seem angry . . . is there something you want that you're not getting?"
	• "You seem afraid . . . do you think something bad is going to happen?"
• Listen	• Try to understand what the patient is saying. "Let me see if I understand correctly." Don't argue. Don't respond to insults
• Agree with the patient	• Do this without lying or furthering a delusion (*see text*)
• Set limits	• Be clear about what is acceptable and unacceptable behavior. Be honest. State positive and negative consequences of behavior. Ask the patient to make a choice
• Offer choices	• "Would you like some medicine to help you calm down?" "Would you like to call someone?"
• Debrief the patient and staff	• After the patient is calm, ask him his reaction to what happened and explain why you took certain steps. Meet with staff as well.

Source: Modified from Fishkind 2002.

If Dr. Fishkind finds a patient banging her fists on a table, he says, "You seem angry . . . is there something you want that you're not getting . . . and do you still want it? Perhaps I can get it for you." If a patient appears frightened, about to flee, he says, "You seem afraid . . . do you feel something terrible is going to happen to you? Can I help you feel safe?" He repeats these statements until the patient appears to relax.

Being with an angry patient will tend to elicit anger or fear in the nurse and anger or fear in the nurse will make it difficult for the nurse to listen. It is crucial, of course, to try and understand what the patient is saying and the nurse needs to overcome his or her anger or fear to be able to listen. Don't argue with the patient. Do not respond to insults with insults.

Agreeing with the patient in some way is important in de-escalation of a potentially violent situation. If the ICU patient on pressor agents wants to go home "right now", you should say, "yes, we need to get you home as soon as possible" or something to that effect. If the delirious, post-op knee replacement patient says that some of the staff are imposters and are trying to kill him, you may say, "we'll do everything we can to make you safe." Although limits need to be set, and although we do not wish to endorse psychotic symptoms, open disagreement usually just riles the already agitated patient.

In setting limits, you must be clear about what is acceptable and what is unacceptable behavior. "We can't allow you to hurt us." In a non-punitive voice, explain the possible positive and negative consequences of behaviors. "If you calm down, we'll get you some ice cream and medicine for your nerves. If you hit us, a security officer will come up to talk with you."

Offering the patient a choice can sometimes be helpful. Perhaps going back to his room for an ice cream or some medication for his nerves. Distinguishing between manipulative anger – often aimed simply at getting more drugs – and anger for other reasons is usually easy because the only thing that will satisfy the drug seeker is drugs.

No matter how hard you try to de-escalate a situation, some patients will still require pharmacological tranquilization and some will even require restraints. When the patient is calm again, you should explain why medication or restraint was necessary and ask about the patient's perspective. When the staff has been traumatized, a debriefing meeting can be healing.

It is beyond the scope of this book to instruct nurses how to defend themselves if actually attacked. We refer the reader to *Managing the Violent Patient: a Clinician's Guide* (Blumenreich and Lewis 1993).

A nurse's recollection of feelings evoked by difficult patients early in her career

The nurse early in his or her career may be so troubled by these patients as to consider leaving the profession. We include here part of an interview with an experienced nurse looking back on her development.

> "In nurses' training, we were taught to accept full responsibility for every aspect of care – physical, mental, spiritual, to take the caretaker role for everything the patient wanted or needed. This seemed natural to me at the time and I went along with it. I took on this role with my peers as well. 'Yes, I can certainly do that,' I said, 'Yes, I can take the most patients,' and so forth. When they said I was wonderful, I thought it lovely, but at some point, it became too much. I began to feel like a martyr.
>
> "For a while I tolerated this feeling. I have a lot of energy. I love nursing. But in the fifth year of my career, I encountered a patient who taught me the need for limit setting. His name was Chad Brandell, a psychopath who'd been in jail. He had lost one leg and was going to lose another if we didn't take immaculate care of it. So I set that as my goal. I would save his leg. I would save this person.
>
> "This involved dressing changes but no matter what I did he ended up lying in stool. His mother and father constantly came to me – I was his primary – begging, 'You've got to help! You've got to!' So I tried one idea after another. Eventually, we discovered he'd been taking laxatives by the handful, which, of course, kept his leg in stool. Later, he began cutting his TPN tubing with scissors. I don't know why he did these things. Maybe it was his way of keeping me in the room, but

when I was there he would say inappropriate things and act out in other ways. He was a troubled soul.

"Each dressing change took about an hour and I did them three times a day. Eventually, I was doing them all day long. I was becoming frantic. Nothing was working. I had to have help but his physicians were totally stymied by him, too. No one wanted to be in his room. Once I took the attending aside – generally a great guy – to talk to him, but instead of expressing sympathy or understanding he said, 'Well, look at it this way. You've learned a lot about dressing changes.' I took umbrage at that.

"Mr. Brandell was in the hospital for about five months. Finally, I *insisted* we do something. We had a family conference run by a physiatrist and rehabilitation psychologist. They told us to 'hand him the bedpan and tell him to sit on it and clean himself up afterwards.' There was no reason he couldn't. The change in his behavior was dramatic. From the bed covered in stool all day, each day, the frequency dropped to approximately one stool in bed every other day. Salvation! I've never forgotten that. We had made a plan and I was determined to see it work.

"Recall that his parents had been begging me to do something, but now that I actually had, they were angry. How could I have the nerve to ask their son to clean up after himself. 'You know,' I told them, 'it's the only thing that works.'

"We followed that plan. After about three more weeks, the patient insisted on going to a nursing home to be allowed to die. He was ill, but he would not allow us to treat him.

"Little by little over the years, I realized that in order to survive, I had to set limits. I've never forgotten how dramatically this patient's behavior changed when he was made to experience the consequences of his own actions. Over the years I also began to realize that it was best to simply tell my peers about what I thought were fair and unfair demands on me. They not only accepted that and didn't hate me for it, but respected me more for saying, in a calm way, what I really felt and thought."

Bibliography

Blumenreich PE. Lewis S. Eds. 1993 Managing the violent patient: a clinician's guide. New York: Brunner/Mazel.

Brayley J. Lange R. Baggoley C. Bond M. Harvey P. 1994 The violence management team. An approach to aggressive behaviour in a general hospital. *Medical Journal of Australia.* 161(4):254–8, Aug 15.

Cameron L. 1998 Verbal abuse: a proactive approach. *Nursing Management.* 29(8):34–6, Aug.

Duncan SM. Hyndman K. Estabrooks CA. Hesketh K. Humphrey CK. Wong JS. Acorn S. Giovannetti P. 2001 Nurses' experience of violence in Alberta and British Columbia hospitals. *Canadian Journal of Nursing Research.* 32(4):57–78, Mar.

Fishkind A. 2002 Calming agitation with words, not drugs. *Current Psychiatry.* 1(4):32–9.

Gatward N. 1999 Managing the "manipulative" patient – a different perspective. *Nursing Standard.* 13(22):36–8, Feb 17–23.

Groves JE. 1978 Taking care of the hateful patient. *The New England Journal of Medicine.* 298:883–7.

Jordheim AE. 1986 What's the best way to handle a sexually aggressive patient? *Journal of Practical Nursing.* 36(5):30–3, Dec.

Kurz JM. 2002 Combatting sexual harassment. *RN.* 65(7):65–8, Jul.

Lawrie B. Jillings C. 2004 Assessing and addressing inappropriate sexual behavior in brain-injured clients. *Rehabilitation Nursing.* 29(1):9–13, Jan–Feb.

Libbus MK. Bowman KG. 1994 Sexual harassment of female registered nurses in hospitals. *Journal of Nursing Administration.* 24(6):26–31, Jun.

May DD. Grubbs LM. 2002 The extent, nature, and precipitating factors of nurse assault among three groups of registered nurses in a regional medical center. *Journal of Emergency Nursing.* 28(1):11–17, Feb.

Minarik P. Leavitt M. 1989 The angry, demanding, hostile response. In *Psychological Aspects of Critical Care Nursing.* Riegel B. Ehrenreich D., Eds. Rockville, Md: Aspen Publishers.

Nield-Anderson L. Doubrava J. 1993 Defusing verbal abuse: a program for emergency department triage nurses. *Journal of Emergency Nursing.* 19(5):441–5, Oct.

Nield-Anderson L. Minarik P. *et al.* 1999 Responding to "difficult" patients. Manipulation, sexual provocation, aggression – how can you manage such behaviors. *American Journal of Nursing.* 99, 27–33.

Philo SW. Richie MF. Kaas MJ. 1996 Inappropriate sexual behavior. *Journal of Gerontological Nursing.* 22(11):17–22, Nov.

Stevenson S. 1991 Heading off violence with verbal de-escalation. *Journal of Psychosocial Nursing & Mental Health Services.* 29(9):6–10, Sep.

Zook R. 1997 Handling inappropriate sexual behavior with confidence. *Nursing.* 27(4):65, Apr.

Chapter 8

The ethics of limit setting

Because the provision of *good* nursing care for some difficult patients requires setting limits on their behaviors – denying them their wishes or even insisting that they do things against their will – we must ask, "Is this ethical?" The question is rhetorical, for how can we provide *good* care that is, at the same time, inimical to the patient's interests, i.e., unethical? Nevertheless, to allay fears that the use of limit setting might compromise the ethical standards of the nurse we dedicate a chapter to the subject. The reader will immediately recognize, however, that our discussion barely touches on the wide ranging and voluminously documented discussions of nursing ethics (Benjamin and Curtis 1986; Parkes 1993; Gerber 1995; Edwards 1996; Warelow 1996; Cahill 1998; Castellucci 1998; Allmark P. 1998; Ketefian and Norris 2002; Weiss *et al.* 2002; Wilmot *et al.* 2002; Leino-Kilpi *et al.* 2003; Semple and Cable 2003; Storch and Nield 2003; Verpeet *et al.* 2003; Park *et al.* 2003; Pang *et al.* 2003; Weiner *et al.* 2003; Zoboli 2004; Nelson 2004; Lemonidou *et al.* 2004; Andrews 2004; Monaghan and Begley 2004).

Four ethical principles

Four generally accepted ethical principles for care of the patient include beneficence, non-maleficence, justice, and respect for patient autonomy (Beauchamp 1994):

- The principle of beneficence means we are to do good for our patients, act to benefit them.
- The principle of non-maleficence means we are to avoid harming our patients.
- The principle of justice means we are to treat all our patients equally and fairly.
- The principle of autonomy means we are to respect our patients' wishes and beliefs; liberty and freedom to act; independence. This presumes that our patients have the capacity to make reasoned decisions about their futures (Edwards 1996).

Day-in and day-out nurses adhere to these principles as a matter of course. Note that some argue that decisions based solely on ethical principles may fail us and that refusing to exercise authority to offer help is "false egalitarianism" (Campbell 1984).

Beneficence vs. autonomy

The most frequently encountered ethical dilemma in dealing with difficult patients occurs when the principles of beneficence and autonomy conflict (Woodward 1998). A nurse's act to benefit a patient without the patient's consent is called paternalism and for decades now has generally been frowned on by the nursing profession (Gerber 1995; Breeze 1998) because of the value placed on the patient's autonomy.

To explain why limit setting against a patient's wishes might not qualify as paternalism or, even if it did, why it might be justified, we must say a few words about the concept of autonomy.

Derived from the Greek, autonomy means self-rule, the ability to think and act independently and voluntarily. Theories of autonomy stipulate that it requires rationality (Breeze 1998) so that a patient with irrational thinking[1] might not be acting with true autonomy. But we must be careful not to judge as irrational a decision we think shows bad judgment. A patient, for example, might wish to forgo chemotherapy that has a very good chance of curing a cancer because of fear of side effects, considerations of cost, estimations of length and quality of life, inconvenient venue of treatment, wish to attend first to other matters, religious beliefs, etc. In such a case we may disagree with the patient's decision but can understand the patient's reasoning. We expect the patient, however, to have the capacity to understand what they are being offered and what are the likely consequences of refusal.

Although the moral philosopher John Stuart Mill (1974) claimed that the only legitimate reason to deny a person his liberty is to prevent harm to others, in the clinical setting "paternalistic" action may well be justified if a person's ability to reason is impaired, if a person will be significantly harmed without intervention, or if the person will likely agree with the intervention after it has occurred (Benjamin and Curtis 1986). A patient may not be be acting with true autonomy if we cannot understand the reasons they give for refusing treatment.

> Mrs. Edith Beardsley, age 83, underwent hip replacement surgery the day before and now, from her bed, is trying to call a taxicab to take her home.
>
> "Mrs. Beardsley, you just had surgery. Perhaps you'd better speak with the doctor before you go home," says her astute nurse, using a gentle tone of voice.
>
> "Leave me alone. Get out of here," replies the ungrateful Mrs. Beardsley.
>
> "Is something wrong? May I help you?"
>
> "Oh, don't play Miss Innocence with me, young lady. I know what you're up to, all of you. You can't keep me here against my will. I know my rights. I'm going home." She picks up the phone again.

Should the nurse help her make the call? That would be respecting her autonomy.

> "Mrs. Beardsley, you seem very upset. What's wrong? Are you in pain?"
>
> "You cannot keep me prisoner here. I want to leave now. Do you understand! Now!"
>
> "Mrs. Beardsley, you can't walk yet. You might fall down again."
>
> "Then get me a wheelchair. I'm leaving."
>
> "I'd like you to stay and speak with the doctor before you go," says the nurse.
>
> "No. I don't want to. You can't make me."

Now, of course, there are a number of reasonable actions the nurse might take but let's allow the nurse to stay in the room a while longer to do a little more assessment of the patient' mental status.

> Recalling that anger and fear emerge together in the amygdala,[2] the nurse asks, "Are you frightened?"
>
> "Wouldn't you be frightened if someone was trying to kill you?"

Mrs. Beardsley has become delusional after an operation and does not have the capacity to make a rational decision on the matter before her.[3] On that basis alone, the principle of autonomy should not apply. Preventing a dislocation of the new hip is called for by the principle of beneficence. She should not be allowed to leave the hospital until it is safe for her to do so.

But what if no delusional content is forthcoming? The patient just wants to go home, that's all. Her judgment appears poor but she is not confused or forgetful.

What if we add ingredients to the case to make a discharge home a recipe for disaster – for example, blood clots, falls, infection, stroke, etc. Might a paternalistic stance be called for after all? Is there such a thing as "autonomy run amok"? (Bellantoni 2003). When does the principle of non-maleficence override the principle of autonomy? What about the patient who does not want to be turned in bed though he is at risk to develop bed sores? We cannot answer these questions out of context, raising them only because nurses are regularly faced with cases that challenge clinical and ethical judgment. We are, after all, simply trying to show why appropriate limit setting is ethical.

> An elderly man is admitted with gastrointestinal bleeding. Although usually quiet and uncommunicative he is at times verbally and physically abusive of staff. His wife has visited occasionally, standing at the doorway, but has not entered his room. With treatment completed and discharge imminent, he demands to be sent home. His wife says this is impossible. She is terrified of him.

At some point, patients with dementia may no longer be able to function autonomously. Surrogates will make decisions for them (Koppelman 2002). Nurses will face ethical dilemmas with these patients (Wilmot *et al.* 2002; Weiner *et al.* 2003).

Let us look at another clinical situation.

> Armand Pleck, 39, a computer programmer whose Crohn's disease has been managed with anti-inflammatory drugs and very high dose narcotics for pain, finally consents to a total colectomy, a procedure he has long feared. His pain is difficult to control post-operatively until the anesthesiologist, sensitized to the patient's high opioid tolerance, greatly increases the continuous infusion rate of morphine administered by the patient-controlled anesthesia machine as well as the size and frequency of the morphine boluses. Mr. Pleck still complains of pain but now sleeps for long periods during the day. He also continually requests the IV lorazepam, diphenhydramine, morphine, or promethazine when their scheduling allows them to be administered "as needed".
>
> He calls the nurse to his room.
>
> "I'm ready for that lorazepam now."

She leaves to get the medication but when she returns he is soundly asleep. He is perfectly still. She counts his respirations, four per minute. She counts for a full two minutes. She shakes him vigorously and he awakens.

"Do you have the lorazepam?"

"Mr. Pleck, I'm afraid I can't give you this right now. Your respiratory rate was very low and this could lower it further."

"My breathing is just fine. I need that medicine now. Dr. Whoosh said I could have it every four hours and the time is up."

"Breathing is very important to your health, you know. If you stop breathing. . . ."

"I won't stop breathing. Now let me have the medicine the doctor ordered."

Granted this is a straightforward illustration of the principle of non-maleficence – give the drug, kill the patient – but the principle is regularly applicable to cases where limit setting is called for.

Let's look at a third scenario.

Mr. Badmouth, in the hospital because of an abscess on the thigh, insists on swearing. This troubles his nurse.

"Hey, I asked you an hour ago for my f-ing medicine. What's taking so long?"

"I'm sorry, Mr. Badmouth, but it isn't due for another 45 minutes."

"Of all the f-ing hospitals I've ever been in, and I've been in a lot, honey, this is the absolute f-ing worst."

"I'm sorry you feel that way. We do want to help you."

"Yeah, right."

"Mr. Badmouth I wonder if you'd be so kind as to stop swearing while you're here. This language makes me uncomfortable."

"I'm the one who's uncomfortable, baby."

"Please don't use curse words. It makes it harder for me to care for you and it upsets the other staff and patients."

"I'm in pain, that's why I'm using swear words, g-damn it."

"I really would appreciate it if you wouldn't curse. Please try not to."

"Oh for crying out loud! Doesn't anyone here understand anything?"

Well, doesn't the patient have right to curse if he feels like it?

"Yeah, I've got a right to curse."

"Stay out of this, would you. We're trying to write a book."

"Yeah, sure."

When patients use bad language in the hospital or clinic the appropriate nursing response cannot be determined simply by asking whether the patient has the right to curse, that is, whether the patient's autonomy must be respected. We must take into consideration the rights of others, the effect on others of the cursing, and also the pragmatic question of what can realistically be expected of the particular offending patient. Sadly, verbal abuse of nurses is common (Lynch *et al.* 2003). Does the above case qualify as verbal abuse? The patient is, after all, cursing the hospital, not the nurse.

Whatever the answer to this question, setting limits to maintain a therapeutic atmosphere for others, to act with beneficence toward others, easily justifies limit setting with Mr. Badmouth.

Joe H., frequently violent and unpredictable, is admitted from prison for a second kidney transplant, the first having failed because of non-compliance. Prison stipulations are that a guard be at his door at all times and that the patient wear ankle cuffs. After the transplant, dialysis is temporarily required for an episode of acute renal failure. This Joe refuses unless certain wishes are granted him – one of which is removal of the ankle cuffs.

Ms. W., a hypercholesterolemic diabetic (HbA1c = 13.7) on chronic benzodiazepines and opioids, is admitted through the Emergency Room in the early morning hours with complaints of nausea, vomiting, and abdominal pain. She said she had just taken insulin but was unable to retain food or fluids. The night shift nurse reports that her 6:00 am blood glucose level is "388 because she has eaten all night after being admitted." For breakfast, Ms. W requests three extra pats of butter and cream for her coffee and cereal, which are proscribed by her hospital diet. She spends her day on the phone, watching television, requesting food, and asking for a cigarette. She rates her head, back, and belly pain as 10 out of 10, demanding narcotics and tranquilizers.

Mr. N. has been using heroin for 15 years and is admitted for repeated abscess formation requiring intravenous antibiotics and dressing changes. He is frequently off the ward smoking at the times of his scheduled treatments.

To limit or not to limit? Beneficence or autonomy? Non-maleficence or autonomy? These are the questions.

Sometimes a patient's behavior becomes so egregious that care cannot be provided by a particular institution; the ultimate in limit setting is the refusal to care for the patient (Lipley 2001). Ethical decision making can be extremely complex in some cases (Zollo and Derse 1997).

Although the reader will doubtless experience situations of ethical ambiguity as regards the use of limit setting, we hope to have demonstrated here that if good care demands it, limit setting is ethical. This is not because care in and of itself is virtuous but because good care is (Allmark 1998).

Bibliography

Allmark P. 1998 Is caring a virtue?. *Journal of Advanced Nursing.* 28(3):466-72, Sep.

Andrews DR. 2004 Fostering ethical competency: an ongoing staff development process that encourages professional growth and staff satisfaction. *Journal of Continuing Education in Nursing.* 35(1):27–33; Jan–Feb.

Beauchamp TL (1994) The "four principle" approach. In *Principles of Health Care Ethics.* Pp 3–12. Gillon R. Ed. Chichester: John Wiley and Sons.

Bellantoni L. 2003 What good is a pragmatic bioethic? *Journal of Medicine & Philosophy.* 28(5–6):615–33, Oct–Dec.

Benjamin M. Curtis J. 1986 *Ethics in Nursing*. 2nd Edn. Oxford: Oxford University Press.

Breeze J. 1998 Can paternalism be justified in mental health care? *Journal of Advanced Nursing*. 28(2):260–5, Aug.

Cahill J. 1998 Patient participation – a review of the literature. *Journal of Clinical Nursing*. 7(2):119–28, Mar.

Campbell AV (1984) *Moderated Love: A Theology of Professional Care*. London: SPCK.

Castellucci DT. 1998 Issues for nurses regarding elder autonomy. *Nursing Clinics of North America*. 33(2):265–74, Jun.

Edwards DS. 1996 *Nursing Ethics: a Principle-Based Approach*. London: Macmillan Press.

Gerber L. 1995 Ethics and caring: cornerstones of nursing geriatric case management. *Journal of Gerontological Nursing*. 21(12):15–19, Dec.

Grossman S. 1997 How can nurses use limit setting to facilitate spinal cord patients' independence? *SCI Nursing*. 14(3):105–7, Sep.

Ketefian S. Norris D. 2002 The recent revision of the Code of Ethics for Nurses with Interpretive Statements (American Nurses Association). *Research & Theory for Nursing Practice*. 16(4):219-21, Winter.

Koppelman ER. 2002 Dementia and dignity: towards a new method of surrogate decision making. *Journal of Medicine & Philosophy*. 27(1):65–85, Feb.

Leino-Kilpi H. Valimaki M. Dassen T. Gasull M. Lemonidou C. Schopp A. Scott PA. Arndt M. Kaljonen A. 2003 Perceptions of autonomy, privacy and informed consent in the care of elderly people in five European countries: general overview. *Nursing Ethics: an International Journal for Health Care Professionals*. 10(1):18–27, Jan.

Lemonidou C. Papathanassoglou E. Giannakopoulou M. Patiraki E. Papadatou D. 2004 Moral professional personhood: ethical reflections during initial clinical encounters in nursing education. *Nursing Ethics: an International Journal for Health Care Professionals*. 11(2):122–37, Mar.

Lipley N. 2001 Turning the tables. Violent or abusive patients can now be banned from NHS treatment. *Emergency Nurse*. 9(8):7, Dec–Jan.

Lynch J. Appelboam R. McQuillan PJ. 2003 Survey of abuse and violence by patients and relatives towards intensive care staff. *Anaesthesia*. 58(9):893–9, Sep.

Mill JS. 1974 *On Liberty*. London: Penguin Books.

Monaghan C. Begley A. 2004 Dementia diagnosis and disclosure: a dilemma in practice. *Journal of Clinical Nursing*. 13(3a):22–9, Mar.

Nelson S. 2004 The search for the good in nursing? The burden of ethical expertise. *Nursing Philosophy*. 5(1):12–22, Apr.

Pang SM. Sawada A. Konishi E. Olsen DP. Yu PL. Chan MF. Mayumi N. 2003 A comparative study of Chinese, American and Japanese nurses' perceptions of ethical role responsibilities. *Nursing Ethics: an International Journal for Health Care Professionals*. 10(3):295–311, May.

Park HA. Cameron ME. Han SS. Ahn SH. Oh HS. Kim KU. 2003 Korean nursing students' ethical problems and ethical decision making. *Nursing Ethics: an International Journal for Health Care Professionals*. 10(6):638–53, Nov.

Parkes R. 1993 Code of ethics for nurses in Australia. *Australian Nursing Journal*. 1(3):28–30, Sep.

Semple M. Cable S. 2003 The new Code of Professional Conduct. *Nursing Standard*. 17(23):40–8; quiz 50–1, Feb 19–25.

Storch JL. Nield S. 2003 Keeping codes current. An ethics program to support nursing practice. *Nursing Leadership Forum*. 7(3):103–8, Spring.

Verpeet E. Meulenbergs T. Gastmans C. 2003 Professional values and norms for nurses in Belgium. *Nursing Ethics: an International Journal for Health Care Professionals*. 10(6):654–65, Nov.

Warelow PJ. 1996 Is caring the ethical ideal? *Journal of Advanced Nursing*. 24(4):655–61, Oct.

Weiner C. Tabak N. Bergman R. 2003 Use of restraints on dementia patients: an ethical dilemma of a nursing staff in Israel. *JONA's Healthcare Law, Ethics, & Regulation*. 5(4):87–93, Dec.

Weiss SM. Malone RE. Merighi JR. Benner P. 2002 Economism, efficiency, and the moral ecology of good nursing practice. *Canadian Journal of Nursing Research*. 34(2):95–119, Sep.

Wilmot S. Legg L. Barratt J. 2002 Ethical issues in the feeding of patients suffering from dementia: a focus group study of hospital staff responses to conflicting principles. *Nursing Ethics: an International Journal for Health Care Professionals*. 9(6):599–611, Nov.

Woodward VM. 1998 Caring, patient autonomy and the stigma of paternalism. *Journal of Advanced Nursing*. 28(5):1046–52, Nov.

Zoboli EL. 2004 [Rediscovering the ethics of care: focus and emphasis in the relationships]. [Portuguese] *Revista Da Escola de Enfermagem Da Usp*. 38(1):21–7, Mar.

Zollo MB. Derse A. 1997 The abusive patient: where do you draw the line?[see comment]. *American Journal of Nursing*. 97(2):31–5; quiz 36, Feb.

Chapter 9

Families

We had intended to call this chapter "Difficult families", modifying the definition of "difficult patient" accordingly, but after reviewing the extensive nursing literature on families decided that a more all-encompassing approach was necessary. Families of difficult patients, after all, may or may not be difficult themselves. Furthermore, families of unproblematic patients may be difficult. We do not intend here to review the broad area of families, their roles, and their assessment (Hanson 1996; Craven and Hirnle 2003), but rather to illustrate some specific areas of concern for nurses caring for difficult patients. We will illustrate some barriers to effective family communication – which is of utmost importance in caring for any patient – describe stressors and emotional responses among families, and discuss gangs and celebrities who have their own special "families".

During a decade of unprecedented debate over which persons may legitimately be called "family" we think it prudent, because it's realistic, to include in this discussion all those who see themselves as family, including close friends. Clearly those with the strongest bonds to the patient will be most deeply affected, and may be co-sufferers (Farkas 1980).

Communication

Nursing communication with families is critical but can be difficult. Davis, Krisjanson, and Blight (2003) identify and illustrate barriers to communication with families. Here we abbreviate their conclusions and refer the reader to their article for first person accounts of the difficulties nurses encounter (Table 14).

Team contributions to family communication problems include, among other things, team conflict, lack of treatment plan, lack of doctor–nurse communication. Work environment factors to communication problems include inadequate space for discussion, acute versus palliative philosophy, excessive workload, and insufficient time. Doctors may not "have" the time either (Hauser and Schwebius 1999).

Such difficulties in communication with families cause frustration, guilt, and a sense of inadequacy in nurses. Davis *et al.* (2003) recommend a renewed focus on team conferences and family meetings, and especially with the legitimization (by the physician?) of the role of the nurse as communicator of the treatment plan, education of nurses in communication skills, and other institutional changes. This approach is being advocated in end-of-life care (Curtis *et al.* 2001).

Table 14 Family factors affecting communication

Factor	Example, illustration, or comment
• Family conflict	• Trying not to take sides is stressful
• Culture–language	• It is difficult to assess what family members understand
• Denial	• The man's death is nigh, but his fiancée keeps talking about the marriage
• Unfamiliarity with the family	• How can you be comforting if you just met the family?
• The family is not fully informed by the physician	• The nurse can't provide the necessary support because the family doesn't understand what is really happening
• Overbearing families or distrustful families	• The family refuses to leave the room for any procedure and is hypervigilant for nursing errors
• Communication among families	• Many relatives pass on information from one to the other so that it inevitably becomes distorted
• Children in family	• It is stressful for nurses when young children are involved but seen as inadequately cared for

Source: Modified from Davis *et al.* 2003.

In some settings, at least, it appears that families more often initiate communication with nurses than the other way around (Walker and Dewar 2001). They may not hold the nurse responsible however:

> "It's nothing to do with the nurses. I know they're run off their feet and it's not really a complaint, what I'm saying is that if I want to find out anything about my mum I have to go and ask, and when you ask you feel a pest because they've got so much on, there's no move towards me (carer)."
>
> (Walker and Dewar 2001)

On the other hand there are "difficult" families that staff avoid as one nurse illustrates:

> "It's not that the relatives want to talk to them [i.e. the staff], it's that these relatives are coming to shout at them, and we had various relatives that we knew were going to come in and start shouting at us. Every day they would stand and shout at us and that is very wearing and you can see why people think 'oh no please', you just want to hide because you're doing a difficult enough job . . . as nurses you're supposed to take all this . . ."
>
> (Walker and Dewar 2001)

In the discussion following this quotation it becomes clear that the nurses felt they must endure this treatment

> ". . . we can't say 'well I'm not speaking to you, go away' because you have to think where is this anger coming from . . . it's about building relationships and if you don't respond to things in a positive way you could damage things so you're trying to be so understanding all the time and that's hard work (qualified nurse)."

The angry family must be engaged, as we have described in other parts of this book, otherwise the nurse's resentment will build, leading to more disengagement and hence more family anger. Families want to feel that information is shared, that they are included in decision making, and that there is a responsive person they can contact when needed (Walker and Dewar 2001). The initial investment of time and patience will pay dividends in later harmony. Family coping styles differ and must be understood (Jens *et al.* 2001).

Sometimes family members and patients fail to communicate with each other (Zhang and Siminoff 2003) to avoid psychological distress or to protect each other or because they believe in positive thinking. The nurse may inquire of individual family members, either separately or in a group, what their understanding is of the clinical situation. The nurse's role as educator of and provider of information to families is well known. It is sometimes complicated when family members disagree among themselves about which of them is entitled to information. In the general hospital the nurse is often the person who must tactfully sort this out.

Families who no longer trust nurses and doctors – if they ever did – are particularly difficult to work with. Their loved one has been managed poorly – either in reality, family perception, or both – at another hospital before being transferred to the current hospital. The patient may now have complex problems – the intensive care unit (ICU) "train wreck" – and may require a long hospital stay with many stressful procedures. After their bad experience at the other hospital, family members are distrustful. They may repeatedly ask a the nurse, "Why are you doing that?" or object to procedures "Don't do that. It upsets him," or refuse to leave the room when asked to do so. They may become extremely angry if, without being properly educated, their wishes are ignored. Of course, behind this anger is the fear of loss of the loved one, the oft-mentioned fight or flight response.

Nursing care of the family in the intensive care unit is an essential and demanding task (Soderstrom *et al.* 2003). When nurses feel that their technical care of the patient supersedes other responsibilities, time demanded by the family can be resented, but when attention to the family is seen as directly helping the patient, time is more easily spent in family communication. Interaction of family members with the same nurse in the ICU was a determinant of family satisfaction (Johnson *et al.* 1998).

Because having a relative in the ICU is often a particularly stressful experience for families, ICU teams studied family satisfaction. In a large Canadian study families were generally satisfied with the care provided, particularly with nursing skill, competence, and compassion and the respect nurses showed to the family and the patient (Heyland *et al.* 2002).

Family stressors and reactions

The stressors families endure are easy to understand. They are physical and emotional. Yates (1999) lists some of them for cancer patients but they apply to families of all seriously ill patients.

Physical stressors include: need always to be available, lack of sleep, exhaustion, disrupted daily routine, unfinished household chores, disruption of plans, disruption of work, and worsening health because of these stressors.

Emotional stressors include: inability to complete chores, resentment, isolation, guilt, sense of loss of control, lack of understanding of the illness, inefficiency, divided loyalty between patient and family, and loss of patience.

Families may also feel guilt because they are in good health, because they feel they should have prevented the illness or detected it sooner, because they cannot treat the patient's discomfort, reduce the nausea or pain, insomnia, and malaise (Wochna 1997).

> Mrs. Green, who lives alone and whose house, by report, is in disarray, is admitted to hospital after fracturing her hip in a fall. She then suffers from alcohol withdrawal and develops aspiration pneumonia. She has no visitors until one day her only son arrives from out of town. He takes up residence in a nearby hotel and is in the hospital from daybreak to bedtime, questioning the nurse about every medication and treatment, hovering at the bedside keen on discovering any fault in the nursing care, needlessly warning the nurse not to hurt his mother during repositioning.
>
> Warren Green had not spoken to his mother for 30 years, a decision he made because of their discordant and painful relationship. Now that she is seriously ill he is assuaging his guilt about her deterioration and his lack of involvement by being a dogged advocate, at the expense, of course, of the nursing staff.

Hospitalized patients around the world are lonely (Gomes and Fraga 1997; Geller *et al.* 1999; Humborstad *et al.* 2001) and nurses are generally pleased to see families present to help comfort these patients. Patient support by families can even improve survival (Christensen *et al.* 1994; Holder 1997). However, nurses can be annoyed by families whose behavior does not conform to their expectations. By recognizing stressors on families, unfair judgment of their behavior may be avoided (Wochna 1997).

> Mr. Oldham is in hospital for chemotherapy of his lung cancer. Day in and day out his wife is at the bedside, her chair parallel to the bed so that both spouse and patient face the wall. She knits. They talk little but when they do her tone of voice is gruff.
>
> "The nurse said you should drink that. So drink it!"
>
> "It tastes so bad, honey."
>
> "Oh for crying out loud. Just drink it, will you."
>
> The nurse thinks, "My goodness, the poor man is going to die within a year and she's talking to him like that." The nurse may or may not later discover the following:
>
> Mrs. Oldham is angry with her husband for getting sick. She had badgered him for years to stop smoking. Now, just as they reach retirement age and were

planning a second honeymoon trip across the Atlantic on the Queen Elizabeth II, he develops lung cancer. They are expecting their third grandchild this month but she will be unable to visit. Her own arthritis is painful and the commute to the hospital each morning is difficult.

Most relatives of seriously ill patients are anxious but anxiety is expressed in individual ways.

Mr. Matloch, a 41-year-old man with a history of AIDS, undergoes an abdomino-perineal resection of an anal carcinoma, develops an agitated delirium for which he is appropriately begun on IV haloperidol, but then develops severe muscle stiffness, fever, and obtundation – neuroleptic malignant syndrome (NMS).

He must be intubated for respiratory failure, probably due to adult respiratory distress syndrome.

His brother Dave spends much time in the intensive care unit. Although propofol is generally effective in keeping the patient's agitation under control, he does awaken from time to time restless or agitated. Dave then impatiently demands the patient immediately be given more sedative. If the patient appears even modestly uncomfortable Dave demands analgesia be immediately administered. Even the expected interval necessary to obtain and administer medications upset him. He complains aloud to the nurse that resources and procedures at "this hospital" seem lacking.

The patient's brother also incessantly asks questions, some of which are quite sophisticated.

"I read on the internet that bromocriptine is used to control the fever. Are you thinking of using it?"

Days pass. The patient remains confused. The blood level of his creatine phosphokinase, however, a measure of muscle damage, has fallen dramatically and muscle tone has improved, though not fully. Dantrolene, a muscle relaxant with the potential to cause liver damage, has been discontinued. A neurologist is now consulted to see if neuroleptic malignant syndrome is still contributing to the patient's ongoing delirium. The neurologist does not think so and agrees that dantrolene should not be reinstituted. Dave argues with her, failing to understand that she is only saying that currently NMS is not a major contributor to the patient's problems. She has not denied that he did, in fact, earlier have NMS.

The patient's intensive care nurse recognized that Dave's intense anxiety was manifested by his incessant questioning – annoying but tolerated – and intolerance of any sign of discomfort in his brother. All his questions were answered. At times she explained that some emergence from unconsciousness and restlessness was actually good for the patient. Note that in this intensive care unit there were no restricted visiting hours, which would have been intolerable for the brother.

The families of critically ill patients require honest information about the patient's condition and treatment. They need to have access to the patient and a sense that their loved one is cared for by the staff (Gavaghan and Carroll 2002).

Consistency of the messages coming from different staff members is important in allaying patient anxiety. Note that Dave had assimilated the idea that his brother was suffering from NMS. He was unable to fully understand what seemed to him a discordant message from the neurologist. The nurse later explained that the neurologist had not denied that the patient *had* suffered from NMS but that he was not now suffering from it.

Engaging, learning from, or simply experiencing families

A fringe benefit of nursing is getting close to and learning from people from all walks of life, being humbled by their strengths and learning from the frailties. How differently each of us reacts to the burden of an ill loved one.

> Opal M., 45, suffering from diabetes mellitus, hypertension, and hyperlipidemia, was being transferred from another unit in the hospital. Morbid obesity had generated severe venous compression ulcers bilaterally, now infected and requiring frequent and extensive, daily dressing changes. Her behavior was proving an obstacle to her recovery. She often refused dressing changes, appropriate activity, physical and occupational therapy. Responding to her frequent and excessive demands for food, her husband brought in boxes of See's candy, whole pies, and cakes. This inimical behavior frustrated the nursing staff. Mr. M. was invited to a unit conference. An appropriate caloric diet, based on patient preferences, was determined, and phone calls for special dietary requests were proscribed. Mr. M. was asked to stop buying treats for his wife.
>
> It was not as if Mr. M. did not acknowledge the problems. Prior to this admission, as he was assisting Opal from the bathroom, she fell on top of him, and both were trapped beneath her walker necessitating a call to the fire department to free them. Yet Mr. M. was very reluctant to deny his wife's wishes. One moment he agreed with the staff to do what he could to hasten her convalescence, the next he expressed anger at the staff for interfering in the couple's usual pattern of behavior.

Contrast this with the story of Nancy C.:

> Her husband Bob, 59, suffering from necrotizing pancreatitis, had been in the hospital for almost a year. During all these months, as he looked death in the eye on the way to another emergent procedure, as new rotations of doctors and nurses again asked her which routines worked best, as she wobbled from worry and fatigue, she never lost her temper, spoke harshly, or gave up hope.
>
> Their daughter's wedding had been planned for his sixtieth birthday but as it became clear he would still be in hospital the venue was changed. His room became the wedding chapel and the hallway became the aisle down which the bride and her attendants walked. Without Nancy's graceful strength and determination Bob would not now be home tending his garden.

Other family tribulations elicit from us wonder:

> An elderly, rural couple drives three hundred miles three times a week so he can be dialyzed. She donates to him a kidney to ease their remaining years together. They then bravely accepted their fate when the kidney failed.

What will the future hold for the 19-year-old athlete who donates a kidney to his grandfather?

A nurse experiences the parents' almost palpable grief as an eye enucleation is planned for their handsome young son. An iron splinter from his shovel gashed his eye as he buried his beloved cat.

The aged Italian woman who speaks little English and does not drive takes a taxi 25 miles each day to sit quietly beside her gravely ill husband.

The young mother of three whose breast cancer has returned.

In the days before ultrasound, a husband leaves the delivery room and does not return during his wife's post-partum stay when the second child is born a girl and not a boy.

Learning about old people from their families; enlisting family help

When patients are old,[1] frail, and confused, lying amidst a tumble of white sheets in a sterile hospital room, we should always turn to their families for stories of more vibrant days, careers, hobbies, talents, adventures, and loved ones.

"My father was one of the most vital men I have ever met. Brilliant and fiercely independent, his wonderful storytelling, sense of humor, and generous heart reflected his Irish heritage. A rancher, state legislator in the House of Representatives, self-educated in law; he was a leader of men. In his late seventies, colon surgery complicated by an anastamotic leak resulted in a stroke and his retirement from public life. Vivid in my mind is the day nursing staff referred to my father as 'elderly'. 'Surely you can't be talking about my father,' rang through my mind and heart. Although, in retrospect, it was an appropriate description, I have since refrained from using that particular term in conversation with my elderly patients' families."

The presence of family can help eliminate restraints and sedatives.

Mrs. Jones, an elegant woman in her eighties, underwent successful abdominal surgery but developed a delirium after meperidine – ill advised in the elderly – had been administered for post-operative pain. She was found in another patient's room, having pulled out her Foley catheter, nasogastric tube, and intravenous line and left them behind. She expressed her paranoia and fear with obscenities. The meperidine was stopped and her son was asked to sit with her until the confusion cleared. Her serene, elegant personality returned.

Family can provide orientation:

An elderly woman was being admitted with a diagnosis of early Alzheimer's disease. When asked about physical activity level, she proudly responded that only yesterday she had walked three miles. With a smile, her son reminded her that it was only because she had gotten lost!

Gangs

Gang violence occurs in large cities around the world (Rosenfeld JV 2002; Kee *et al.* 2003; Leon-Carrion and Ramos 2003; Ochicha *et al.* 2003; Paglia and Adlaf 2003). These references are from Australia, Canada, Indonesia, Nigeria, Spain, and the U.K. Most medical and nursing articles about gangs are derived from study in cities in the United States and doubtless there are differences in gang culture from Seattle to Singapore to Saskatoon, but gangs everywhere serve one function – to offer a place of belonging, a family.

Grossman and McNair (2003) discuss attributes of American gangs which are applicable elsewhere. Nursing staff must understand the three R's of gang thinking – *reputation, respect, and retaliation* – in order to understand the gang member patient.

For the individual within the gang and for the gang itself to "survive" they must have a *reputation* for toughness, lest they be bullied or attacked. The individual and the gang, always conscious of how their actions affect their reputation, may be brutal to maintain or enhance it. Their bravado is more than show.

Gang members demand *respect* for themselves, their family members, their territory, and for the gang itself. Other gangs may show disrespect by gesturing, staring, or writing graffiti on a rival's territory.

Although a gang member may leave the area after he has experienced disrespect, he will return later, perhaps weeks later, along with fellow members, to *retaliate* to restore his reputation

Grossman and McNair (2003) make the following suggestions for emergency room staff:

- Act professionally, radiate confidence.
- Treat a gang member's possessions with respect. His bandanna may be your crystal vase.
- Separate rival gangs.
- Be alert for signs of tension: aggressive posture, loud or profane speech, and restlessness.
- Remove gang graffiti immediately from hospital walls.
- Minimize eye contact and avoid hand signals.
- Keep ample distance between you and the patient.
- Don't allow a potentially violent person between you and the door.
- Have security guards search potentially violent patients and remove weapons. Keep guards near. Do not take a weapon from a patient. Ask him to put it down and then call security or the police.
- Remove potentially dangerous items – such as chairs, intravenous poles, and hot drinks – from the examination rooms before the patient enters.
- Don't wear personal items such as stethoscopes, scissors, or jewelry that could be used as a weapon against you.
- If you're attacked, tuck your chin down to protect the carotids if you're choked. If you're bitten, push toward the patient and plug his nose.

- Don't argue, cry, whine, fight, or run away if a weapon is shown. Try to alert others to the imminent danger and to determine what the attacker wants. Don't try to wrestle the weapon away – it's time to bargain. Use your words. Words don't bleed.

Once the gang member has been admitted to the hospital, problems may continue. Morrison, Ramsey, and Snyder (2000) describe the experience of nurses working in a large city hospital serving a largely poor, minority population. They describe problematic behaviors of young men, often drug dependent, often violent, and their family members, friends, and acquaintances. They describe concretely how sufficient positive attention, structure, and limit setting, especially if instituted early, can improve patients' behavior.

"Celebrity patients, very important persons (VIP's) and potentates"

The heading of this section is the title of an article by Groves, Dunderdale, and Stern (2002). We discuss these patients here because their entourages may be considered families of sorts even if they are retainers or attendants.

Celebrities are people[2] whose "lives interest the public most when something bad has happened to them." The principal problem created for the nurse caring for the rock star, movie star, king, senator, oil magnate, Nobel laureate, Olympian, or mass murderer is having to work under intense and often public scrutiny. This is distracting and stressful, and can impair judgment.

The well-prepared hospital will try to shield the staff by assigning one person to deal with the media, but staff members are still likely to feel the heat of the spotlight, to be badgered with questions, and possibly be stung by criticism by members of the retinue.

> Johnny Lust, of Johnny Lust and the Thrusters, a rock star known for public displays of vulgarity, is nevertheless extremely popular. He is admitted to hospital with a closed head injury after falling from the back of a flat bed truck while displaying his buttocks to a crowd of fans. His manager, Mr. Pfau, only slightly less exhibitionistic, holds forth in front of the hospital entrance making veiled threats about what might happen to the doctors and nurses should anything happen to this gift to world music. Unfortunately there is no one spokesperson assigned. Before the news cameras, the neurologist, neurosurgeon, internist, differ slightly from each other in the terms they use to describe the patient's condition, prognosis, and treatment plan. Seeming contradictions are magnified by Mr. Pfau. The doctors become irritated with each other.
>
> Meanwhile the nurse is offered a large sum of money from a tabloid paper to give her view of things. Johnny's attorney, bodyguard, spouse, manager, masseur, secretary, and fellow musicians don't like the way she is treating their boy and have no qualms letting her know it. Meanwhile Mr. Pfau and Johnny's spouse each demand that the other receive no updates from the doctors. Shortly afterwards the neurosurgeon is designated the public spokesperson, and using the tactic suggested by Groves, Dunderdale, and Stern, threatens to quit the case unless both Johnny's

girlfriend and manager can be updated, and unless everyone leave the room when the nurse is working with the patient.

VIP's — a term attributed to Sir Winston Churchill — command special privilege, prestige, and influence in a particular area, inspiring awe in those working in that domain. The VIP that nurses are most likely to encounter is a physician from the same medical center. Physicians treating this VIP physician, fearful of making an error, may order unnecessary tests or, on the other hand, wishing to spare their colleague distress, may forego appropriate though uncomfortable tests. The VIP's entourage may be as problematic as the celebrities but the spotlight may be less hot.

The last category is the potentate, persons who think they are special by virtue of their wealth or position. For the staff they are only difficult patients with money and may have their retinues as well.

A well-coordinated team approach, with designation of a hospital spokesperson, one or two patient spokespersons, and clear lines of communication, can reduce stress for all involved.

Concluding remarks

Because of their special relationship with the patient, families are generally "stronger" than any individual physician or nurse. If we can engage them to be our partners everyone benefits.

Bibliography

Christensen AJ. Wiebe JS. Smith TW. Turner CW. 1994 Predictors of survival among hemodialysis patients: effect of perceived family support. *Health Psychology*. 13(6):521–5, Nov.

Craven RF. Hirnle CJ. 2003. Families and their relationships. In *Fundamentals of Nursing: Human Health and Function*. 4th Edn. Philadelphia: Lippincott Williams and Wilkins.

Curtis JR. Patrick DL. Shannon SE. Treece PD. Engelberg RA. Rubenfeld GD. 2001 The family conference as a focus to improve communication about end-of-life care in the intensive care unit: opportunities for improvement. *Critical Care Medicine*. 29(2 Suppl):N26–33, Feb.

Davis S. Kristjanson LJ. Blight J. 2003 Communicating with families of patients in an acute hospital with advanced cancer: problems and strategies identified by nurses. *Cancer Nursing*. 26(5):337–45, Oct.

Farkas SW. 1980 Impact of chronic illness on the patient's spouse. *Health and Social Work*. 5: 39–46.

Gavaghan SR. Carroll DL. 2002 Families of critically ill patients and the effect of nursing interventions. *Dimensions of Critical Care Nursing*. 21(2):64–71, Mar–Apr.

Geller J. Janson P. McGovern E. Valdini A. 1999 Loneliness as a predictor of hospital emergency department use.[erratum appears in *J Fam Pract* 1999 Dec;48(12):1002]. *Journal of Family Practice*. 48(10):801–4, Oct.

Gomes LC. Fraga MN.1997 [Illness, hospitalization and anxiety: an approach to mental health]. [Portuguese] *Revista Brasileira de Enfermagem*. 50(3):425–40, Jul–Sep.

Grossman V. McNair M. 2003 Emergency: gang members in the ED. *American Journal of Nursing*. 103(2):52–3, 2003 Feb.

Groves JE. Dunderdale BA. Stern TA 2002. Celebrity patients, VIP's, and potentates. Primary care companion. *Journal of Clinical Psychiatry*. 4(6):215–22.

Hanson SMH. 1996 Family assessment and intervention. In *Family Health Care Nursing: Theory, Practice, and Research*. Hanson SM. and Boyd ST. Eds Philadelphia: F. A. Davis.

Hauser W. Schwebius P. 1999 [Four minutes for the patient and one minute for the families. Physician–patient–family communication in medical departments]. [German] *Psychotherapie, Psychosomatik, Medizinische Psychologie*. 49(5):168–70, May.

Heyland DK. Rocker GM. Dodek PM. Kutsogiannis DJ. Konopad E. Cook DJ. Peters S. Tranmer JE. O'Callaghan CJ. 2002 Family satisfaction with care in the intensive care unit: results of a multiple center study. *Critical Care Medicine*. 30(7):1413–18, Jul.

Holder B. 1997 Family support and survival among African-American end-stage renal disease patients. *Advances in Renal Replacement Therapy*. 4(1):13–21, Jan.

Humborstad OT. Omenaas E. Gulsvik A. 2001 [Consumer surveys among hospitalized patients with lung disease]. [Norwegian] *Tidsskrift for Den Norske Laegeforening*. 121(9):1066–9, Mar 30.

Jens GP. Chaney HS. Brodie KE. 2001 Family coping, styles, and challenges. *Nursing Clinics of North America*. 36(4):795–808, viii, Dec.

Johnson D. Wilson M. Cavanaugh B. Bryden C. Gudmundson D. Moodley O. 1998 Measuring the ability to meet family needs in an intensive care unit. *Critical Care Medicine*. 26(2):266–71, Feb.

Kee C. Sim K. Teoh J. Tian CS. Ng KH. 2003 Individual and familial characteristics of youths involved in street corner gangs in Singapore. *Journal of Adolescence*. 26(4):401–12, Aug.

Killam P. 2003 Maintain relationships with challenging families. *Nurse Practitioner*. 28(6):15, Jun.

Leon-Carrion J. Ramos FJ. 2003 Blows to the head during development can predispose to violent criminal behaviour: rehabilitation of consequences of head injury is a measure for crime prevention. *Brain Injury*. 17(3):207–16, Mar.

Lipson JG. Dibble SL. Minarik PA. 1996 *Culture and Nursing Care. A Pocket Guide*. San Francisco, Ca: UCSF Nursing Press, Univ. of Calif San Francisco.

Morrison EF. Ramsey A. Synder BA. 2000 Managing the care of complex, difficult patients in the medical-surgical setting. *MEDSURG Nursing*. 9(1):21–6, Feb.

Ochicha O. Mohammed AZ. Nwokedi EE. Umar AB. 2003 A review of medico-legal deaths in Kano. *Nigerian Postgraduate Medical Journal*. 10(1):16–18, Mar.

Paglia A. Adlaf EM. 2003 Secular trends in self-reported violent activity among Ontario students, 1983–2001. *Canadian Journal of Public Health*. 94(3):212–17, May–Jun.

Rosenfeld JV. 2002 Gunshot injury to the head and spine. *Journal of Clinical Neuroscience*. 9(1):9–16, Jan.

Soderstrom IM. Benzein E. Saveman BI. 2003 Nurses' experiences of interactions with family members in intensive care units. *Scandinavian Journal of Caring Sciences*. 17(2):185–92, Jun.

Walker E. Dewar BJ. 2001 How do we facilitate carers' involvement in decision making? *Journal of Advanced Nursing*. 34(3):329–37, May.

Wochna V. 1997 Anxiety, needs, and coping in family members of the bone marrow transplant patient. *Cancer Nursing*. 20(4):244–50, Aug.

Yates P. 1999 Family coping: issues and challenges for cancer nursing. *Cancer Nursing*. 22(1):63–71, Feb.

Zhang AY. Siminoff LA. 2003 Silence and cancer: why do families and patients fail to communicate? *Health Communication*. 15(4):415–29, 2003.

Chapter 10

Communicating with doctors – the difficult and the easy

In Hindu mythology an avatar is an incarnation of a god, a god in the flesh as it were. In Chapter 6 a nurse fearlessly approached Dr. Avatar with clear knowledge of what she wanted, but he was a mere mortal, the name given him only an allusion to the arrogance and inapproachability of some physicians. Such arrogance may be fostered by the respect accorded physicians historically; by their unconscious view of death as the enemy; and, especially, by physicians' knowledge. It may be manifested by lack of respect and good manners towards nurses as well as others (Berger 2002). We, the authors, are hardheaded enough to know that some of the avatars you deal with professionally are incorrigible. We believe, though, that physician overwork is more likely to interfere with communication than arrogance (Rutter *et al.* 2002) and that good nurse–doctor relationships are the rule rather than the exception. The whole issue is complicated when we speak of male and female roles in different cultures.

You will be unable to care properly for your patient, the difficult and the not so difficult, if you cannot enlist the physician's assistance. At the very least the physician must convey to you the plan for caring for the patient. Which infection is being treated? For how long? Any special worries the physician has? And so forth. At the least, you, in return, must be able to communicate to the physician how the patient is responding to treatment and which patient behaviors are obstacles to the provision of good nursing care.

The literature contains hundreds of articles on the nurse–doctor relationship, relatively few of which are based on research. Sweet and Norman (1995), working in the United Kingdom, review some of this literature from a sociologic perspective. We will not endeavor to describe in detail the roots of the difficulties that some nurses and doctors have had with each other, but will describe a familiar pattern of interaction which, though less prevalent than it was 40 years ago, can still be observed today.

The doctor–nurse game

In 1966 Hildegard Peplau described a changing relationship of nurse to doctor from subservient to collaborative. A form of that collaboration or that interpersonal communication was examined the very next year by Stein (1967), who wrote of a common pattern of communication between nurse and doctor which he dubbed the "doctor–nurse game". If both the nurse and doctor play it well, both of them win. The team functions effectively, the doctor gains a valuable consultant in the person of the nurse, the nurse gains self-esteem and satisfaction in her[1] work. If they fail at the game, the physician is resented and his life made more difficult by a nurse not fully engaged in assisting him. The nurse who fails to play her role as consultant is seen as a dullard and is excluded from involvement.

The rules of the game are as follows. (1) There must be no open disagreement. (2) The nurse must make recommendations without appearing to do so. (3) The physician must request recommendations without appearing to do so. In this manner neither physician nor nurse commit themselves to a position until a sub rosa agreement has been reached between them. In this way open disagreement is avoided.

A round of the game might appear as follows.

> The setting: Level 10, a surgical ward with specialization in gastrointestinal disorders. Nurse Good, caring for Mr. Allooch, a 35-year-old man with acute alcoholic pancreatitis, approaches the surgical resident, Dr. Stitch, who has just examined the patient and sees no significant clinical change.
>
> "Dr. Stitch, Mr. Allooch is in more pain today. Last admission he took much more morphine to keep him comfortable."

The first statement is a straightforward communication of fact. Less openly it appears to be a recommendation.

> "How much morphine did he get last time?"

He is asking for a recommendation without appearing to do so.
No harm appears to have occurred in this scenario. Let's look at another.

> Mr. Matloch, a 41-year-old man with a history of AIDS, alcohol dependence, IV amphetamine use, and chronic pain treated for months with high doses of narcotic analgesics undergoes an abdominoperineal resection of an anal carcinoma. Post-operatively his pain is very difficult to control even by the anesthesiologists. He moans and yells, receiving high dose IV hydromorphone, lorazepam, transdermal fentanyl, and briefly at one point, even ketamine. Since he has also become delirious the anesthesiologists appropriately add IV haloperidol to his regimen.
>
> The day after surgery the nurse notes that the patient's muscle tone is increased. This is particularly noticeable when he is turned from side to side. It is hard to flex and extend his arms and legs.
>
> "Doctor Gray, Mr. Matloch seems rather stiff to me."
>
> In her twenty years in the intensive care unit she's never seen anything quite like this and she's worried that there was an occult pathological process occurring.
>
> "Yes, he seems that way to me, too. I'm not sure what he was like before. We'll keep an eye on him."
>
> The patient's intermittent periods of agitation resolve after a few more doses of IV haloperidol but he becomes unresponsive and even more rigid.
>
> The nurse calls Dr. Gray.
>
> "Mr. Matloch's agitation has resolved but . . ."
>
> "Good! Fever down?"
>
> "No, not really, no. He's very stiff."
>
> The doctor pauses, "Hmm . . . I'll come by tonight to look at him."

"He's very stiff, Dr. Gray."

He examines the patient that night and is also worried. He discontinues the narcotics and stops the haloperidol. He does not elicit recommendations and the nurse does not offer them. She doesn't think the doctor is doing enough but doesn't know what the right thing to do would be. She does not want confrontation though ideas sometimes emerge from dialogue, from confrontation, from disagreement.

A day goes by before the doctor realizes that this is a case of neuroleptic malignant syndrome, a rare, but potentially fatal complication of major tranquilizer drug use, characterized by severe muscular rigidity, hyperthermia, and autonomic disturbances (Susman 2001; Antai-Otong 2003; Waldorf 2003).

Let's change the scenario somewhat.

"Doctor Gray, Mr. Matloch seems rather stiff to me."

"Yes, he seems that way to me, too. I'm not sure what he was like before. We'll keep an eye on him."

"I'm really quite worried. I've never seen anything like this. Is there anything else we should be doing?" Though she doesn't know what exactly to recommend, the nurse speaks out about her discomfort, putting aside any qualms she may feel about belittling his knowledge or judgment.

"Yes, I suppose we'd better stop the haloperidol and reduce the narcotic dose."

By speaking up now rather than later the nurse has prompted the physician to act, shortening the patient's exposure to haloperidol, the offending agent, by many hours and significantly improving the patient's course.

Her asking, "Is there anything else we should be doing?" is, in essence, a recommendation for more action. An experienced physician working collaboratively might have said, "I'm not sure. What do you think?" The doctor–nurse game has now been replaced with direct communication.

Blickensderfer (1996) advises that nurses simply refuse to play the doctor–nurse game by communicating assertively, honestly, directly and, of course, respectfully. She outlines a series of proposals to further collaboration between doctors and nurse.

Ineffective communication between the nurse and doctor and, worse still, hostility in communication between them is obviously detrimental to the function of the healthcare team. In two papers Davidhizar and Dowd (2001, 2003) discuss the establishment and maintenance of good communication between the nurse and other healthcare professionals, especially doctors. The following discussion is largely derived from these papers.

Awareness of one's own reactions to people

At the outset the nurse should recognize in herself unpleasant emotions evoked by interactions with a doctor who may remind her of another person in her life with whom interactions were unpleasant. Such a reaction is termed countertransference. For example, if the nurse had an uncle with a walrus mustache and a loud voice who used to come over to the house and tease her for being clumsy, and later in life she encounters in the hospital a physician with a walrus mustache and a loud voice, she may react to his comments as teasing and may become angry though he meant no harm. Davidhizar and Down suggest the nurse ask herself, "Does the doctor remind me of someone in my past. . . . a parent, teacher, or other authority figure . . . or perhaps even another doctor?" A reaction to others as if they were an important figure from the past is sometimes termed countertransference because of the transfer of feelings related, for example, to a parent to, again for example, an attending physician. Positive feelings need no attention, but if the physician is in fact benign yet the nurse is angry or defensive because of countertransference, then the nurse must do a little self-analysis.

Nurses should be aware of their own areas of sensitivity. A nurse who fears his or her minority culture is not respected may interpret benign comments as disrespectful of that culture; a nurse insecure about his or her technical skills may interpret benign comments as suggestions of incompetence; a female nurse who believes all male doctors expect subservience may interpret benign comments as derogatory of women in general.

Word choice for better communication

Davidhizar and Dowd suggest avoiding the phase "You should" since it may be interpreted by the physician as authoritarian. Even the physician consultant who has been asked by another physician to give advice may avoid this phrase, especially when unsure of the proper course or of the requesting physician's underlying assumptions. The consultant might say, "*Please consider*" ordering a TSH or doing an ultrasound, for example. Nevertheless, direct communication is efficient and we think you should say "you should" when appropriate. You can even combine terms:

> "Dr. Avatar, I really think you should consider ordering some haloperidol for Mr. Palooka. He's still thinks he's in a boxing match and keeps punching at the staff."

You must be able to make suggestions even to those seemingly unreachable physicians.

> "Were you planning to give us some direction?"
> "Do you think Mr. Godzilla could benefit by a tranquilizer?"
> "When do you feel the family should be called in?"

The staff development firm Development Dimensions International, Inc. also stresses the importance of work choice on our impact on others.

Instead of "Why did you do that?" consider "What do you think happened?"

Instead of "That will never work," consider "What will we need to do to make this successful?"

Instead of "It's not my responsibility," consider "What part of this *am* I responsible for?"

Being prepared before calling the physician

Only sedated saints are uniformly gracious when wakened in the middle of the night by someone who demands their help but can't tell them what for.

Table 15 Before calling the physician get your ducks in order

- Assess the patient
- Review the chart to identify which physician is the appropriate one to call
- Know the admitting diagnosis
- Read the most recent progress note and the assessment from the nurse on the prior shift
- While speaking with the physician have available: the chart; the list of allergies and medications; IV fluids; laboratory and X-ray results; intake and output data; and recent vital signs
- Have formulated in your mind or on paper what you would like to see done
- Phrase recommendations thoughtfully, for example: "Do you think we should . . ."
- Be prepared to explain why you think your recommendation makes sense

The nurse calling during the day should also have the pertinent data at hand. Although this is common sense we thought we would underscore it by making a table (Table 15).

Illustrations of nurse–physician communication

Mrs. Inoa, a native of Hawaii, is admitted with irreversible liver disease four days prior. She is not a candidate for a liver transplant. Her condition suddenly worsens with anuria, decreased level of alertness, hypotension, and diminished oxygen saturation of hemoglobin. Sitting at her bedside and seeing her mother's deterioration, her daughter is frightened. The nurse calls the appropriate physician with the clinical information and asks, "Do you think we should establish 'do not resuscitate' orders?" The physician responds by coming directly to the ward to meet with the nurse and the daughter for an emotion-laden discussion of the patient's condition. Four hours later the patient dies peacefully with her family at the bedside.

Of course, life being what it is, not all cases are characterized by good nurse–physician communication.

Mr. Troy, admitted with severe pancreatitis, has been in hospital now for three weeks with complications of pseudocyst, clotting abnormalities, respiratory difficulty, and pain. Towards the end of the shift the nurse notes bright red drainage from an abdominal drain that had been placed by the interventional radiologist earlier in the day. Although vital signs had changed little, the seasoned gastro-enterology nurse is fully aware that this is a sign of danger. She speaks with the intern on-call and makes recommendations, "Do you think we should type and cross? Should we transfer the patient to the intensive care unit?"

"No, let's just observe the patient," says the intern. The patient's condition worsens and the nurse makes a second call, this time speaking with the resident who concurs with the intern.

Mr. Troy now develops bright red bleeding per rectum. The nurse makes a third call. The form of her recommendation changes: "Dr. Lingam, this patient is now in imminent danger. My shift is over but I will not leave until you come to see the patient now."

The patient is now transferred to the intensive care unit where he receives ten units of packed red blood cells. The resident spends the night there.

A repeat scenario is unnecessary between this nurse and physician, but from a patient's perspective this is a difficult way to improve the team's communication.

Time and place for communication

If you anticipate an adverse reaction from a difficult doctor you should[2] speak with the physician when there will be some privacy. If you publicly address Dr. Avatar with your concern or request, he may feel this is a sign of disrespect, even insubordination.

Confrontation

Confrontation, the direct expression of disagreement between two parties, does not include in its definition snarling, screaming, or cursing from either party. In other words we can confront people calmly and politely.

"Please, don't leave your chewing gum on the bedpost overnight."[3]

"Dr. Thunder, please lower your voice a bit, you're frightening me."

"I'm sorry Mrs. Chimney, but we don't allow smoking here."

Act diplomatically and non-defensively if you decide to confront a physician. Your goal is to resolve a problem. You should not be drawn into an emotional argument. You may consider beginning your confrontation with "I feel that." You cannot be told that, "No, you don't feel . . .". On the other hand, a physician believing that he or she is acting on the facts, that is scientifically, may disregard your feelings.

You may wish to confront condescension or irrational anger directed at you by a physician.

"Dr. Thunder, I really felt bad when you raised your voice with me this morning. I gave the prn morphine as you had ordered it. Mr. Blue had been receiving it all along for days with no reduction in respiratory rate until this morning. I am following your instructions as best as I can. Please tell me how I could have predicted what happened and I will watch out for it from now on."

Avoid reacting with anger

Anger and fear, fight or flight, are flip sides of the same adrenaline-linked response (Jansen *et al.* 1995). In confrontation with another person we may have one or the other reaction. Anger is a natural response in a conflict and also when one is being treated unfairly or feels trapped because of lack of power in the relationship. You will feel anger in some interactions with physicians. You heart may pound. You may feel tremulous. Your voice may quaver. You need not, however, overtly display that anger by raising your voice, cursing, or crossing your arms across your chest and frowning. Recall that vocal or visual display of emotions tend to elicit those same emotions in others (Heilman and Gilmore 1998). We tend to be happy around happy people, sad around sad people. In fact, your anger in an interaction with a physician may have been triggered by that same physician's anger toward you. The reason you should try not to express your anger is that it may elicit anger in the physician. Communication between two angry people is likely to be inefficient.

If you cannot reduce the intensity of your anger in a situation, you had best wait until it subsides before confronting the physician (or anyone else, for that matter). Do not respond immediately unless you can muster a calm tone of voice, a non-defensive facial expression and physical posture. Then you may wish to provide objective information calmly.

Again from Davidhizar and Dowd (2001):

> "I have the equipment you need ready and I'll get it for you now. Your loud voice is making me feel nervous, and I do want to do a good job helping you."

Enculturation of nurses and doctors

An experienced nurse of many years recalled for us some of her experiences as a student nurse:

> "In 1964 a respected surgeon spoke at one of our required lectures, 'Acceptable behavior towards physicians'. Even after all these years I clearly recall one of his requests: 'When a physician enters, please stand as a sign of respect and as an indication that you are there to assist.' Mercifully, this attitude no longer prevails – at least not in Canada and the United States. Since nurses no longer sit, the advice is irrelevant and for the most part physicians and nurses have learned the value of a collaborative rather than a subservient relationship."

There remain, of course, modern day medical and nursing cultural barriers to effective collaboration between doctors and nurses (Blickensderder 1996).

Doctors are trained to solve problems independently whereas nurses are trained to work collaboratively.

Their goals may differ at times as when the nurse is preparing a patient for a comfortable and dignified death and the doctor is still trying to reverse the pathogical process.

They spend little time talking to each other even to resolve their differences. Some doctors respond to a nurse's questions as if their authority were being questioned or express annoyance when they are called after hours because the nurse is worried about a change in a patient's condition.

Changing the culture

The call from nurses for a more collaborative approach to patient care is increasingly heard (Henneman *et al.* 1995). Enmon and Demitropoulos (2004) describe the formation of a unit-based interdisciplinary focus team to improve communication among hospital staff. Dechairo-Marino *et al.* (2001) describe a method of studying the effects of formal programs to foster nurse–physician collaboration.

A nurse's recollection:

> "A turning point in my career occurred many years ago. I had just admitted a patient from the emergency department who had many confusing symptoms. The resident entered and after examining the patient, he asked what I thought the diagnosis was and what corrective action we might take together. This was the beginning of my journey down the path of nurse–physician collaboration. Encouraging this journey was a Nurse–Physician Collaboration Committee which helped explore our patients' clinical trends, learn their treatment plans, and establish rapport and communication between disciplines."

It might be argued that the gold standard of nurse–physician communication is found in interdisciplinary rounds (Curley *et al.* 1998; Halm *et al.* 2003), yet physicians and nurses are under time pressure to care for and treat with complex therapies acutely ill, unstable patients. Some nurses are uncomfortable rounding with physicians preferring to "just get the work done." Some physicians fail to see the importance of coordinating efforts. We believe the benefits of rounding merit the initial expenditure.

> The nurse clinical advisor is approached one afternoon by a frustrated physician. A serum and a urine sodium level had been ordered the previous day. Blood had been drawn that morning for the serum level but urine had not been collected until several hours after furosemide had been administered. The two sodium levels could no longer be compared. The measurement would have to be repeated. How easily this scenario could have been avoided if the plan of care had been discussed in the patient's room with the nurse present.

Such coordination is even more important in providing good care for the manipulative, drug-seeking patient.

> Mr. Beal has been hospitalized with an infected abscess at the site of a heroin injection. He relentlessly asks for more and more narcotic analgesic. Nurses exhausted by his badgering begin to avoid him. A physician called in the middle of the night gives the following order, "May have meperidine 100 mg IV, one dose." This exception powerfully rewards Mr. Beal's attemps to get higher doses of narcotics and, from a nurse's perspective, make him insufferable.

Alternatively:

> Nurse Sharp recognizes the pattern of manipulative behavior and arranges a patient care conference with the nurses and physician caring for Mr. Beal. The appropriate narcotic dose is calculated for the patient's comfort and to prevent withdrawal.

Together the nurse and physician explain to the patient the plan of care which will be strictly adhered to unless the patient's physical condition changes. After a day of testing the nurses, the patient is no longer insufferable.

We have seen this approach work again and again.

Physicians from different cultures

Barriers to effective communication may arise if a male physician from a culture where women are indeed expected to be subservient does not learn that his new environment demands a more collaborative approach toward females in general and nurses in particular. A female nurse from a matriarchal culture may bristle at the male physician who feels his authority is absolute. Unfortunately, all we can offer is a supplication for patience and understanding. Simple differences in style of communication can be major obstacles to teamwork.

A nurse offers the following recollection:

"Miss M. was admitted with a gastrointestinal hemorrhage complicated by IV drug use. She was hostile and threatening to the staff and frequently, after her 'visitors' left, exhibited periods of rage and irrational behavior to the point that hospital security had to be called. In the nurse's view, the resident physician in charge of the case, who was born and raised in China, ignored their fears and concerns, spent little time with the patient, and became further and further removed as the nurses became more and more desperate for solutions in dealing with Miss. M.

"A nurse arranged for an objective physician[4] uninvolved with the case to conduct a round table discussion. This meeting has always stood out in my mind because of its effectiveness. We were each asked honestly to state what we felt were the problems. After heartfelt discussion we were each asked what we had gained from the meeting. The foreign resident felt that his response to the situation was in large measure due to his enculturation where verbalization over conflict was minimized, but now, on hearing the nurses' accounts of the situation, he understood why the nurses felt unsupported. I personally realized how my communication could have been more direct and effective. I had entered the meeting feeling that I could not work with this particular physician on another case. By the end of the meeting I knew we could once again be part of a collaborative team and for the remainder of his residency at the hospital we were.

"From this meeting I learned the power of good communication, how it can change the most difficult scenarios, how people from different cultures approach communication differently but can learn how to be effective in the new culture they find themselves in."

Disruptive physicians

Harmony at work is a wonderful thing, probably even lengthening our lives. Caring effectively for patients supports that harmony. Good relationships with our colleagues supports that harmony.[5] The disruptive physician may dash all hopes of harmony.

There is no generally accepted definition of a "disruptive physician" but disruptive behaviors are generally agreed on. Note that our definition of difficult patient can easily be modified to define a "difficult physician", one whose behavior is an obstacle to the provision of good nursing care.

Disruptive behaviors of physicians include (Piper 2003):

- Sexual harassment
- Racial or ethnic slurs
- Intimidation and abusive language
- Persistent lateness in responding to call
- Threatening or abusive language
- Degrading and demeaning comments
- Profanity or other grossly offensive language
- Threatening or intimidating physical contact
- Public derogatory comments about quality of care
- Inappropriate medical record entries concerning quality of care
- Idiosyncratic requirements on staff that have nothing to do with better patient care.

This is so blatant. How can physicians engaging in even a few of these behaviors be allowed to stay on staff? Piper explains some of the obstacles to confronting such physicians effectively.

First they are often clinically excellent, highly intelligent, and have a considerable following. The disruptive physician from the old guard may have himself been a chief of staff and prominent member of the medical community. The young disruptive physician may be well liked because of energy, passion, and motivation. Though both share a low threshold for explosive behavior towards staff, it is often extremely difficult to muster both objective evidence of transgressions and persons willing to support a confrontation. Nurses are deterred from reporting disruptive behavior for fear of "retaliation, concerns about a report's impact on future relations, and the belief that 'nothing ever changes'." They are also worried about confidentiality, peer pressure, and potential legal ramifications (Rosenstein 2002).

Piper outlines the institutional steps that can help confront such physicians, a listing of which here is irrelevant. The general topic of the disruptive physician, however, is, of course, relevant to the care of difficult patients if these physicians are responsible for their medical management. Clearly nurses alone will be unable to resolve the behaviors of such physicians. They are generally considered impaired physicians and must be dealt with by the chief executive of the organization with the support of other high level administrators.

Physicians who are generally not disruptive do occasionally have outbursts of temper when orders they consider crucial to good patient care, especially for unstable patients, are not carried out promptly or as ordered. They may also be annoyed when called by a nurse who does not have the pertinent patient data immediately available. A nurse might well respond in the same manner. In the high-pressure arena of hospital care such occasional temper flares continue. Nurses respond adaptively to occasional verbal abuse by physicians viewing the abusing physician as a person with a problem and holding themselves as undeserving of such treatment (Manderino and Berkey 1997).

Here is a vignette from a now experienced nurse about an early experience:

"For several years I worked with a brilliant surgeon whose frequent disruptive outburst frightened me and, at times, humiliated me. Because I was young and new in my position, his behavior took me totally off guard. One of his preferences was having the patient's family wait in the patient's room so he could inform them regarding the results after surgery.

"One day a particular family was unable to wait. He appeared on the ward and was furious that his wishes had been ignored. He began yelling at me. He kicked the garbage can across the room and shoved the patient's bed against the wall. As he fumed down the hall, I was finally able to explore the situation objectively. His actions were inappropriate. They had nothing to do with me or my handling of the situation. I did not have to tolerate such disrespect and lack of maturity. I resolved never to endure such treatment again. With that inner resolve and without my saying a word came the most amazing result. Dr. T. never treated me that way again in the remaining years we worked together.

"It is important that we nurses and physicians accept responsibility for our occasional errors, tardiness, and personality quirks. We are human. However, our errors do not justify intimidation, harassment, demeaning comments and a host of other inappropriate actions. We should not endure them."

Concluding remarks

Nurses have become more assertive, autonomous, and accountable (Taylor-Seehafer 1998) over the entire history of the nursing profession. More and more are also engaged in collaborative relationships with physicians. Nurses still have legitimate grievances, but we are saddened when, for example, we hear a nurse at a distinguished nursing lecture belittling physicians as generally inept and using them as the butt of cruel jokes, for this illustrates lingering discord between the professions.

It would be difficult or impossible to identify from the literature in which countries the nurse–physician relationship flourishes and in which it does not, but there are significant differences from hospital to hospital, city to city, district to district, and country to country (Hojat *et al.* 2003). Communication between doctor and nurse may have its regional idiosyncrasies but it has always been vital to the well-being of patients everywhere. Because nurses in the general hospital are present with difficult patients for hours at a time but physicians are not, nurses usually are most affected by patient's troubling behaviors. We hope that the reader has found here practical suggestions to communicate with and engage physicians in the care of patients.

For those nurses dealing with incorrigible physicians we hope this chapter points the way to some resolution.

Bibliography

Antai-Otong D. 2003 Adverse drug reactions associated with antipsychotics, antidepressants, and mood stabilizers. *Nursing Clinics of North America.* 38(1):161–76, Mar.

Atkinson JH Jr. 1982 Managing the violent patient in the general hospital. *Postgraduate Medicine.* 71(1):193–7, 200–1, Jan.

Barrere C. Ellis P. 2002 Changing attitudes among nurses and physicians: a step toward collaboration. *Journal for Healthcare Quality.* 24(3):9–15; quiz 15–6, 56, May–Jun.

Berger AS. 2002 Arrogance among physicians. *Academic Medicine.* 77(2):145–7, Feb.

Blickensderfer L. 1966 Nurses and physicians: creating a collaborative environment. *Journal of Intravenous Nursing.* 19(3):127–31, May–Jun.

Curley C. McEachern JE. Speroff T. 1998 A firm trial of interdisciplinary rounds on the inpatient medical wards: an intervention designed using continuous quality improvement. *Medical Care.* 36(8 Suppl):AS4–12, Aug.

Davidhizar R. Dowd S. 2001 How to get along with doctors and other health professionals. *Journal of Practical Nursing.* 51(1):12–4; quiz 15–7, Spring.

Davidhizar R. Dowd S. 2003 The doctor–nurse relationship. *Journal of Practical Nursing.* 53(4):9–12, Winter.

Dechairo-Marino AE. Jordan-Marsh M. Traiger G. Saulo M. 2001 Nurse/physician collaboration: action research and the lessons learned. *Journal of Nursing Administration.* 31(5):223–32, May.

Enmon P. Demetropoulos S. 2004 Bringing talk to the table. *Nursing Management.* 35(3):50–2, Mar.

Gjerberg E. Kjolsrod L. 2001 The doctor–nurse relationship: how easy is it to be a female doctor co-operating with a female nurse? *Social Science & Medicine.* 52(2):189–202, Jan.

Greenfield LJ. 1999 Doctors and nurses: a troubled partnership. *Annals of Surgery.* 230(3):279–88, Sep.

Halm MA. Gagner S. Goering M. Sabo J. Smith M. Zaccagnini M. 2003 Interdisciplinary rounds: impact on patients, families, and staff. *Clinical Nurse Specialist.* 17(3):133–42, May.

Heilman KM. Gilmore RL. 1998 Cortical influences in emotion. *Journal of Clinical Neurophysiology.* 15(5):409–23, Sep.

Henneman EA. Lee JL. Cohen JI. 1995 Collaboration: A concept analysis. *Journal of Advanced Nursing.* 1995;21:103–9.

Hojat M. Gonnella JS. Nasca TJ. Fields SK. Cicchetti A. Lo Scalzo A. Taroni F. Amicosante AM. Macinati M. Tangucci M. Liva C. Ricciardi G. Eidelman S. Admi H. Geva H. Mashiach T. Alroy G. Alcorta-Gonzalez A. Ibarra D. Torres-Ruiz A. 2003 Comparisons of American, Israeli, Italian and Mexican physicians and nurses on the total and factor scores of the Jefferson scale of attitudes toward physician–nurse collaborative relationships. *International Journal of Nursing Studies.* 40(4):427–35, May.

Jansen AS. Nguyen XV. Karpitskiy V. Mettenleiter TC. Loewy AD. 1995 Central command neurons of the sympathetic nervous system: basis of the fight-or-flight response. *Science.* 270(5236):644–6, Oct 27.

Kramer M. Schmalenberg C. 2003 Securing "good" nurse/physician relationships. *Nursing Management.* 34(7):34–8, Jul.

Larson E. Hamilton HE. Mitchell K. Eisenberg J. 1998 Hospitalk: an exploratory study to assess what is said and what is heard between physicians and nurses. *Clinical Performance & Quality Health Care.* 6(4):183–9, Oct–Dec.

Lockhart-Wood K. 2000 Collaboration between nurses and doctors in clinical practice. *British Journal of Nursing.* 9(5):276–80, Mar 9–22.

Manderino MA. Berkey N. 1997 Verbal abuse of staff nurses by physicians. *Journal of Professional Nursing.* 13(1):48–55, Jan–Feb.

Mason DJ. 2002 MD-RN: a tired old dance. *American Journal of Nursing.* 102(6):7, Jun.

Peplau H. 1966 Nurse–doctor relationships. *Nursing Forum.* 5 (1), 60–5.

Piper LE. 2003 Addressing the phenomenon of disruptive physician behavior. *Health Care Manager.* 22(4):335–9, Oct–Dec.

Rosenstein AH. 2002 Original research: nurse–physician relationships: impact on nurse satisfaction and retention. *American Journal of Nursing.* 102(6):26–34, Jun.

Rutter H. Herzberg J. Paice E. (2002) Stress in doctors and dentists who teach. *Medical Education.* 36(6):543–9, Jun.

Sperling RL. 2001Communicating with physicians. *Home Healthcare Nurse.* 19(8):463, Aug.

Stein L. 1967 The doctor–nurse game. *Archives of General Psychiatry.* 16:699–703.

Susman VL. 2001 Clinical management of neuroleptic malignant syndrome. *Psychiatric Quarterly.* 72(4):325–36, Winter.

Sweet SJ. Norman IJ. 1995 The nurse–doctor relationship: a selective literature review. *Journal of Advanced Nursing.* 22(1):165–70, Jul.

Taylor-Seehafer M. 1998 Nurse–physician collaboration. *Journal of the American Academy of Nurse Practitioners.* 10(9):387–91, Sep.

Verschuren PJ. Masselink H. 1997 Role concepts and expectations of physicians and nurses in hospitals. *Social Science & Medicine.* 45(7):1135–8, Oct.

Waldorf S. 2003 AANA journal course. Update for nurse anesthetists. Neuroleptic malignant syndrome. *AANA Journal.* 71(5):389–94, Oct.

Willis E. Parish K. 1997 Managing the doctor–nurse game: a nursing and social science analysis. *Contemporary Nurse.* 6(3–4):136–44, Dec.

Woodham-Smith, C. 1951 *The Life of Florence Nightingale 1820–1910.* New York: Whittlesey House.

Chapter 11

The nurse and the dying patient

We have defined the difficult patient as one whose behavior presents an obstacle to the provision of good nursing care. Why then include a chapter in this book on the dying patient? Is there behavior inherent in the process of dying that is a barrier to the provision of good nursing care? Dying patients may, of course, prove difficult in the same ways that other patients may prove difficult, but we have described these behaviors elsewhere. Although dying, like aging, or like living, is a process rather than a behavior, a dying patient may elicit stress in nurses that is, indeed, an obstacle to the provision of good nursing care. Dying patients as a group may not fit our definition of difficult patients, but caring for them and their families can be stressful so we have decided to dedicate a chapter to the subject of the nurse and the dying patient.

Death anxiety

The fear of death – one's own or someone else's – and the avoidance of thoughts of death or exposure to death in pictures, reading, and everyday life, has been termed death anxiety[1] (Neimeyer 1994). Contrasting mental sets include neutral acceptance of death as an inevitable part of life, positive acceptance of death as a step into a happy afterlife, or acceptance of death as an escape from pain and suffering. The presence of death anxiety in nurses may, in part, determine what sort of nursing practice they choose. Hospice nurses, for example, may, in general, have less death anxiety than emergency room nurses (Payne *et al.* 1998).

Death and dying are widely recognized as sources of nursing stress (Watson and Feld 1996; Lenart *et al.* 1998; Rooda *et al.* 1999; French *et al.* 2000; Timmins and Kaliszer 2002). Working with dying patients and their families may rekindle nurses' own past griefs and anticipatory grief, as well as sensitize them to their own mortality (Worden 1982). Working with dying patients may threaten an individual's sense of "power, mastery, and control" (Rando 1984). Unresolved or complicated grief among nurses working with dying patients may be associated with despair, social isolation, and somatization (Feldstein and Gemma 1995).

Whatever areas of specialization a nurse has chosen, she or he will eventually be faced with dying patients, anticipatory grief, bereavement of family members, and death. In these circumstances nurses with death anxiety will be more stressed than their colleagues.

How does one reduce or eliminate it? The first step is to become conscious of our own mortality and of any anxiety that may be associated with it. Saunders and Valente (1994) list a series of exercises to help accomplish this:

- "Ask yourself 'Is today a good day to die?'" Consider why or why not.
- Find a quiet place and visualize all the details around your deathbed, your dying, and your death.
- Write a will and an epitaph.
- Talk about your expectations of death and afterlife.

Besides anxiety over our own mortality, existential anxiety, we may ask ourselves: Are we re-experiencing an unresolved grief? Are we anticipating the death of someone close to us? Is there something in our experience that makes us feel particularly vulnerable? It may help to try writing down our thoughts, talking to a friend or therapist. People who have suffered traumatic loss may be at particular risk for complicated grief reactions (Rynearson 2001).

Grief

Though studies of the human response to profound loss do reveal certain common reactions, it is misleading to speak of "stages" of grief because not all who mourn take the same path from "painful separation to personal restoration" (Neimeyer 2000; Worden 1982). Furthermore the circumstances of death influence the reaction to the loss. An unexpected loss or loss by violence is different than the loss of someone whose death has long been expected (Rynearson 2001). After the publication of Kubler-Ross's *On Death and Dying* (1969) many novices expected that the dying would go through one "stage" after the next in succession: denial, anger, bargaining, depression, and acceptance. Another conceptualization describes phases of mourning: shock, yearning, disorganization, and reorganization (Bowlby 1973; Parkes and Weiss 1983). Another conceptualization (Worden 1982) describes the tasks of mourning: accepting the reality of the loss; experiencing the pain of grief; adjusting to new roles, demands, and opportunities; and finally withdrawing emotional energy from the deceased and investing it in another relationship.

In his classic study of grief after the Coconut Grove Nightclub fire of 1942 Lindemann (1944) described manifestations of acute grief, which Worden (1982) categorizes as:

- *Feelings* such as sadness, anger, guilt and self-reproach, anxiety, loneliness, fatigue, helplessness, shock, yearning, numbness.
- *Physical sensations* such as hollowness in the stomach, chest tightness, throat tightness, over-sensitivity to noise, de-personalization, shortness of breath, weakness, dry mouth.
- *Cognitions* such as disbelief, confusion, preoccupation, sense of the departed's presence, fleeting hallucinations, both auditory and visual.
- *Behaviors* such as sleep disturbance, appetite disturbance, absent-mindedness, social withdrawal, dreams of the deceased, searching or calling out, sighing, crying, visiting places that are reminiscent of the deceased or avoiding reminders of the deceased, treasuring items that are reminiscent of the deceased.

Grief is the experience of loss. Mourning is the process of change that occurs after the loss. We cannot review here the theories of grief and bereavement except to note that it has generally been accepted that depression is inevitable after a loss, that lack of distress suggests pathology, that it is necessary to work through the loss (grief work), and eventually to relinquish the attachment to the deceased (Lindstrom 2002). This view is not accepted by all the experts. Bonnano and Kaltman (1999) refuted the notion that grief work was beneficial, that depression was inevitable, or that ties to the deceased need be cut. Lindstrom (2002), admitting there are conflicting views and too little knowledge, suggests a middle ground about the best way to mourn, writing that neither a compulsive working through nor a determined avoidance of the emotions and thoughts of grief is in order, that they can be accepted but let pass. The bereaved should get involved in everyday life, and eschew excessive disclosure that may drive people away. Nor, according to Lindstrom must the bereaved sever emotional ties with the deceased.

Nurses' grief

Nurses become attached to their patients and grieve with the families at their deaths (Feldstein and Gemma 1995; Marino 1998; Kelly *et al.* 2000). The stress of grief for the nurse is diminished if she believes she has helped the patient have a good death: a death with minimal distress,[2] a death with the opportunity to say goodbye and make amends, a death that seems natural. More difficult is the grief following suicide or unexpected death. An atmosphere tolerant of the discussion of death and the availability of support groups for nurses does help nurses cope (Saunders and Valente 1994; Lenart *et al.* 1998; Brosche 2003). Simply permitting nurses to talk with each other about dying patients at the time of shift change, nursing handover or sign out, can be helpful (Hopkinson 2002). Curricula for teaching about grief and bereavement (Matzo *et al.* 2003) will help future nurses.

Unfortunately, in the fast-paced modern hospital it is often difficult to find time to spend with dying patients and their families or even with other staff. A nurse related this vignette:

> "One day shortly after the shift change report, a patient had a cardiac arrest and expired. With no time to experience any relationship with this patient, I simply did the necessary paperwork. I was working with a young student nurse that day and as I marched on to the next four acutely ill patients she stopped me with tears in her eyes and asked, 'Could we stop a minute and discuss what just happened?' It took me back to many past experiences and the importance of discussion, of making time to resolve shock, grief, and sadness."

Painful emotions

Emotions evolved as communication between animals (Darwin 1872). As we have written elsewhere, if you are with a sad person you will tend to become sad and if you're with an angry person you will tend to become angry (or frightened). And so it is with the other emotions as well. It is no surprise then that many people tend to avoid people displaying anger. The response to sadness is more variable: it may be avoidance if people do not wish to become sad, or approach if they choose to provide comfort and support.

Tears have formed in the corners of John Trueblood's eyes. His children have just left his hospital room after a meeting with the doctor to discuss the progression of his metastatic tumor. He is alone now, clearly visible from the hallway. Mr. Trueblood knows he's dying. Do his tears reflect sadness, anger, fear, guilt, or another emotion? His nurse, Frank Bond, sees him, waves, and walks by. He'll return in a few minutes. How Frank approaches the patient depends on Frank's personality, training, and on John's personality and situation.

A dying patient, in a poignant and frequently cited letter to a nursing journal, asked, "Is it because I am a student nurse, myself, or just a human being, that I sense your fright? And your fear enhances mine. Why are you afraid? I am the one who is dying" (Anonymous 1970).

Earlier in the letter the patient noted, "You *slip*[3] in and out of my room, give me medication and check my blood pressure." The anxious nurse in such situations will distance herself emotionally, avoid sensitive topics, focus on the purely technical, and spend less time with the patient (Payne *et al.* 1998).

Anger is also difficult to face.

Mark, a handsome, athletic 21-year-old college student was admitted for a surgery on a rapidly growing abdominal cancer. The promise and dreams of his future, he learned, were to end in four to six weeks. When his oncologist suggested that he and his family take a cruise together to share the time remaining, he became so angry that the oncologist felt their relationship was no longer therapeutic and signed off the case. Mark explored every possible treatment, traveling out of the country for medical opinions and treatments. He was readmitted to the hospital six weeks later, where he died.

We suspect that avoidance of dying patients is, in most cases, not due to death anxiety, or even avoidance of troubling emotions, but rather insecurity about what to say or how to provide emotional comfort (McGrath *et al.* 1999).

Broaching the topic of death with the patient

Emily M., age 45, an inscrutable expression on her face, is in bed as her nurse, Kathy O., enters. She has terminal ovarian cancer and has been admitted to hospital for the third episode of small bowel obstruction in a month and a half.

"Good morning, Emily," says, Kathy. Emily nods.

After getting her vital signs Kathy asks, "May I sit here for a moment?"[4] indicating a folding chair near the bed. Emily nods.

"How are you doing?"

"Okay."

"So, Emily, may I ask what's on your mind this morning?"

"Oh, you know. Getting home soon. The kids are a handful for Fred."

"Mmm."

There is a pause[5] then Emily speaks again. "I wonder if I'll be able to go back to work."

Kathy knows the gynecologic oncologist has explained to Emily and her husband that there is no cure, that palliative care may improve quality of life, and that most patients at this stage of illness do not live longer than six months.

"What has your doctor told you about your illness?"

"Oh, you know, that I've got cancer and he's going to treat it."

"Is it serious?"

"Oh, yes, it's serious."

"Did he say how serious it is?"

"Well, it's spread and it's serious. Doesn't she tell you these things?"

"Oh, we talk, of course, but I'd much rather hear your understanding of your illness. Patients can get so much information from their doctors that it's hard to sort out sometimes. It can be a little too much. You say it's serious?"

"I've been in the hospital twice this month."

"Could you die from this illness?"

"Yes." Emily's expression is unchanged.

Kathy has now broached the topic of dying with a patient in a hospital, not a hospice, who is clearly dying and who, it seems, has not yet come to terms with her existential situation. Now consider two of many responses open to Kathy.

Response A:

"Well, I'd like to hear more about this if it's alright with you. I'll be back a little later in the day to chat. Can I get you anything now before I leave?"

Response B:

"Do you ever think about that possibility?"

"I try not to."

"Oh, tell me about that."

It is unnecessary for the reader to pick the "correct" response since the additional information necessary to make a choice is only available to the nurse standing in Kathy's shoes, who at the moment happens to be Kathy. She may have been moving towards this conversation slowly for weeks and sense that this is now the time to pursue it. She may be unable to pursue it at this time because she must first attend to other seriously ill patients. Furthermore, either of them might be the "correct" choice, that is continuing the conversation now or continuing the conversation later.

We believe that broaching the subject of dying with the dying patient who has not expressed himself on the subject is almost always necessary at some time or another to assess whether or not the patient would benefit by talking about it. Many patients will benefit by the opportunity to express their emotions about dying with a nurse who knows how to listen. There are also a substantial number of patients who may not wish to talk about death (Dean 2002). One patient, a psychiatrist wrote, "What I find interesting is how I can spend most of my time not thinking about my prognosis. Is this denial or wisdom? . . . Most of us prefer ignorance about how our sausage was made" (Rifkin 2001). Clearly each patient is an individual with individual needs.

As we noted, the most frequent cause of discomfort in talking to the dying patient probably arises from a sense of inadequacy for the task. McGrath *et al.* (1999) quote some of the nurses in their study:

"But never did I talk to them about their feelings about death and dying. I wanted to, I knew I should, but I couldn't. I felt lost for words."

"[Patient] often tells me she is scared – scared of her future and her death. I have no answer for her. I do not know how to respond."

In almost every case the prognosis, including the information that the disease is incurable and the time short, must initially be conveyed to the patient by the physician, not by the nurse. Even when the nurse knows for certain that the physician has told the patient his condition is terminal, the nurse must not assume that the patient has heard the information, much less assimilated it. This is where assessment comes in as illustrated in the dialogue between Kathy and Emily.

Asking the patient what the doctor has said and what it means to the patient is one way to begin to discover what the patient understands and feels. Encourage the patient to elaborate by asking her to tell you more. Respect the patient's right to remain silent. Find the right time to do the assessment.

Let us present a few brief patient–nurse dialogues:

"Am I going to die?" asks the dying patient.
"Yes, your cancer has spread."

"Am I going to die?" asks the dying patient.
"There's always hope."

"Am I going to die?" asks the dying patient.
"I'm not sure what you're asking me. Please tell me more."

Following this last dialogue – the one we recommend – the nurse might ask any of the following questions.

"What has the doctor told you?"
"What is your understanding of your condition?"
"What is your family's understanding of your condition?"
"How do you feel about this?"
"What's the most difficult part of all this?"
"What subject would most likely bring tears to your eyes if you discussed it?" (*Most frequently it is separation from family, burden to family, or the family's grief.*)
"Can you talk with me a little about this?"
"Do you have questions about your situation?"
"This is make-believe, but if you had an envelope containing the exact date of your death, would you open it?"
"What is the scariest part of this for you?" ("the saddest part, the angriest part, the part you feel most guilty about. . . .")

It is sometimes a mistake to launch an answer to a question whose depths have not been plumbed. There is no substitution for knowing the patient, but knowing the patient takes time. If some of this time has been in intimate contact – during bathing, hair combing, etc. – it will be easier for the patient to express emotions. When that begins suggests a hospice nurse, "Just shut up and listen."[6]

Nurses' small talk and chattiness are sometimes criticized as avoidance of painful subjects, but they are part of normal interactions and part of making the hospital humane and tolerable (Dean 2002).

The grieving spouse in the hospital setting

Hampe (1975) studied the needs of the grieving spouse in the hospital setting. Though the study took place 30 years ago, with a small and specific socioeconomic sample, it was detailed with hundreds of hours of taped interviews and is still relevant today. Some of the identified needs follow and in parentheses the percent of participants expressing these needs:

- The need to be informed of the spouse's condition (100%).
- The need to be helpful to the dying spouse (74%).
- The need to be informed of the impending death (74%).
- The need to be with the dying person (63%).
- The need for comfort and support of family members (41%).
- The need for assurance of the comfort of the dying person (33%).
- The need to ventilate emotions (32%).
- The need for acceptance, support, and comfort from health professionals (15%).

In this study, needs were only partially met. These needs have been incorporated into care plans to orient and reassure the spouse regarding the patient's comfort, to arrange for daily updates on the patient's condition, to allow the spouse to be with and care for the patient, and to provide supportive listening (Dracup and Breu 1978; Youll 1989).

Czerwiecz (1996) noted in her study that the patient's physical comfort was the families' prime concern, whereas their biggest complaint was that they weren't kept informed of the patient's condition. It is difficult to know which of a nurse's many actions are valued by the family and which are unnoticed. The relationship with the family is the most important factor in the family's satisfaction with nursing care and that relationship takes time to establish. The same sorts of assessment questions asked of patients can profitably be asked of families as well.

Our personal histories and reactions to patients

Are we having trouble accepting a particular patient's stance towards dying? A nurse, with a loss of her own in the background, describes her difficulty supporting a terminal patient's refusal to accept his condition.

"Providing care for my sister in her home the last five weeks of her life made the impending loss more bearable. She was dying of breast cancer at 49. I was determined to provide for her wish to die at home and felt empowered with my nursing experience to create an environment of support, peace and tranquility. We reminisced about the glorious freedom of our youth, the pride of family, of jobs well done, of challenges faced and overcome and of the deep love and respect we always shared. One beautiful autumn afternoon I will always remember. Her canary was singing and I massaged her feet as we talked. She smiled and said, 'You know, this is just the most perfect day; and the only thing wrong is that I am dying.'

"Always a strong, committed person, she had made the decision to allow death to progress naturally – after surgery and chemotherapy had failed. She ate until she could no longer lift the spoon to her mouth. Her only cross words were spoken when I tried to feed her when she was no longer able to feed herself. Though dehydration at the end of life is not painful, it was near unbearable to see her as the days wore on without food or water.

"When she became confused the last two weeks, I felt the deep pain of losing her companionship and the fatigue of being up at night to catch her wandering. I felt guilty that life was still ahead for me and that my life had seemed much easier than hers. I was mystified why this wonderful, gifted, brilliant and compassionate woman had to die so young and leaving her daughter motherless. And, although I am generally a calm and reasonable person, I became terribly unnerved by the thought of the hearse driving up to her home and taking her away. In the end, she spent her last 24 hours in the hospital.[7]

"Sometime later I cared for a patient whose attitude bothered me. Jim's adult years had been unproductive. He had been in and out of jail and had several children he did not support. Though he had a terminal illness and his dying had been hastened by years of bad choices, he felt entitled to every possible aggressive treatment to prevent his death. I compared this narcissistic patient's choice with that of my sister who had dedicated her life to helping others and remained totally unselfish even in death. When I discussed my unease with my manager her response immediately put it in perspective: 'But that was your sister's choice – this is Jim's.' Sometimes the hardest part of caring for the dying is reminding yourself, every patient and every family member is different. It's not about you."

Discussion with a pediatric hospice nurse

A nurse who provided in-home pediatric hospice care had no death anxiety nor was she distressed at the process of the child's dying because, as she put it, children did not suffer existential anxiety. Children did not struggle with the questions such as "Have I led a good life?" or "Have I done all I should have done?" Her job was to reduce suffering – not to rescue either patient or family – and to help carry out the medical regimen prescribed by the doctor. She might provide comfort, for example, by teaching that the child's screaming at and struggling against the administration of eye drops was easily overcome by having the child lie supine with eyes closed, putting the drops in the corner of the eyes, and then having the child open the eyes.

She helped the parents, whose intimacy had been disrupted by the presence of the dying child, by asking how they had met.

She prepared them for the death of the child by explaining that "we all clear our throats a hundred times a day" and that when the child is totally relaxed the little fluid in the throat would gurgle. The so-called death rattle was not a sign of pain. She had the parents provide as much care as possible. Why should someone else bathe the child if the parents could do it?

She was, of course, sad when the child died but if she had contributed to a good death she felt rewarded. Nurses manage their own sadness best when they know they have "helped a patient die a good death" (Saunders and Valente 1994).

Bibliography

Anonymous 1970 Death in the first person. *American Journal of Nursing* 70(2):336.

Bonanno GA. Kaltman S. 1999 Toward an integrative perspective on bereavement. *Psychological Bulletin*. 125(6):760–76, Nov.

Bowlby J. (1973) *Separation: Anxiety and Anger*. New York: Basic Books.

Brosche TA. 2003 Death, dying, and the ICU nurse. *Dimensions of Critical Care Nursing*. 22(4):173–9, Jul–Aug.

Czerwiecz M. 1996 When a loved one is dying: families talk about nursing care. *American Journal of Nursing*. 96(5):32–6, May.

Darwin C. 1872 *The Expression of Emotions in Man and Animals*. London: Murray.

Dean A. 2002 Talking to dying patients of their hopes and needs. *Nursing Times*. 98(43):34–5.

Dracup KA. Breu CS. 1978 Using nursing research findings to meet the needs of grieving spouses. *Nursing Research*. 27(4):212–16, Jul–Aug.

Faulkner KW. 1997 Talking about death with a dying child. *American Journal of Nursing*. 97(6):64, 66, 68–9, Jun.

Feldstein MA. Gemma PB. 1995 Oncology nurses and chronic compounded grief. *Cancer Nursing*. 18(3):228–36, Jun.

French SE. Lenton R. Walters V. Eyles J. 2000 An empirical evaluation of an expanded Nursing Stress Scale. *Journal of Nursing Measurement*. 8(2):161–78, Fall–Winter.

Gagne FL. Robichaud-Ekstrand S. 1995 [How to intervene effectively with a dying patient]. [French] *Canadian Nurse*. 91(2):47–51, Feb.

Hampe SO. 1975 Needs of the grieving spouse in a hospital setting. *Nursing Research*. 24(2):113–20, Mar–Apr.

Hopkinson JB. 2002 The hidden benefit: the supportive function of the nursing handover for qualified nurses caring for dying people in hospital. *Journal of Clinical Nursing*. 11(2):168–75, Mar.

Kelly D. Ross S. Gray B. Smith P. 2000 Death, dying and emotional labour: problematic dimensions of the bone marrow transplant nursing role?. *Journal of Advanced Nursing*. 32(4):952–60, Oct.

Kubler-Ross, E. 1969 *On Death and Dying*. New York: MacMillan.

Kulbe J. 2001 Stressors and coping measures of hospice nurses. *Home Healthcare Nurse*. 19(11):707–11, Nov.

Lenart SB. Bauer CG. Brighton DD. Johnson JJ. Stringer TM. 1998 Grief support for nursing staff in the ICU. *Journal for Nurses in Staff Development*. 14(6):293–6, Nov–Dec.

Lindemann E. 1944 Symptomatology and management of acute grief. *American Journal of Psychiatry*. 101:141–9.

Lindstrom TC. 2002 "It ain't necessarily so" [.] Challenging mainstream thinking about bereavement. *Family & Community Health*. 25(1):11–21, Apr.

Marino PA. 1998 The effects of cumulative grief in the nurse. *Journal of Intravenous Nursing*. 21(2):101–4, Mar–Apr.

Matzo ML. Sherman DW. Lo K. Egan KA. Grant M. Rhome A. 2003 Strategies for teaching loss, grief, and bereavement. *Nurse Educator*. 28(2):71–6, Mar–Apr.

May C. 1995 "To call it work somehow demeans it": the social construction of talk in the care of terminally ill patients. *Journal of Advanced Nursing*. 22(3):556–61, Sep.

McGrath P. Yates P. Clinton M. Hart G. 1999 "What should I say?": qualitative findings on dilemmas in palliative care nursing. *Hospice Journal*. 14(2):17–33.

Neimeyer RA. 1994 *Death Anxiety Handbook*. Washington: Taylor and Francis.

Neimeyer RA. 2000 Grief therapy and research as essential tensions: prescriptions for a progressive partnership. *Death Studies*. 24(7):603–10.

Parkes CM. Weiss R. 1983 *Recovery from Bereavement*. New York: Basic Books.

Payne SA. Dean SJ. Kalus C. 1998 A comparative study of death anxiety in hospice and emergency nurses. [see comment]. *Journal of Advanced Nursing*. 28(4):700–6, Oct.

Rando TA. 1984 Grief, dying and death: clinical interventions for caregivers. Champaign, Ill: Research Press.

Rifkin A. 2001 Is it denial or wisdom to accept life threatening illness?. [Letter] *British Medical Journal*. 323(7320):1071, Nov 3.

Rooda LA. Clements R. Jordan ML. 1999 Nurses' attitudes toward death and caring for dying patients. *Oncology Nursing Forum*. 26(10):1683–7, Nov–Dec.

Rynearson EK. 2001 Retelling Violent Death. Philadelphia: Brunner-Routledge.

Saunders JM. Valente SM. 1994 Nurses' grief. *Cancer Nursing*. 17(4):318–25, Aug.

Timmins F. Kaliszer M. 2002 Aspects of nurse education programmes that frequently cause stress to nursing students – fact-finding sample survey. *Nurse Education Today*. 22(3):203–11, Apr.

Timmins F. Neimeyer RA. 2000 *Lessons of Loss. A Guide to Coping*. Center for the Study of Loss and Transition. Memphis, Tenn.

Volker DL. 2003 Assisted dying and end-of-life symptom management. *Cancer Nursing*. 26(5):392–9, Oct.

Watson P. Feld A. 1996 Factors in stress and burnout among paediatric nurses in a general hospital. *Nursing Praxis in New Zealand*. 11(3):38–46, Nov.

Worden JW. 1982 *Grief Counseling and Grief Therapy: a Handbook for the Mental Health Practitioner*. New York: Springer Press.

Youll JW. 1989 The bridge beyond: strengthening nursing practice in attitudes towards death, dying, and the terminally ill, and helping the spouses of critically ill patients. *Intensive Care Nursing*. 5(2):88–94, Jun.

Chapter 12

Nurses and stress

We include in this book a chapter on stress, not only because difficult patients may stress nurses but because a nurse already under stress may have particular difficulty caring for patients who add to this burden. Perhaps this chapter will prove simply to be a consciousness-raising exercise because every nurse with any experience is acquainted with stress and has tried to reduce it (McVicar 2003).

Hans Selye (1985), who established the modern study of stress, defined it as a non-specific or generalized physiological response to a variety of environmental stressors. The familiar phrase, the hypothalamic–pituitary–adrenal axis,[1] derives from his work (Haddad *et al.* 2002; Bailey *et al.* 2003). For Selye, stressors may be emotional as well as physical, and the stress response is not necessarily undesirable. We will use the term stress here, however, in a more restricted, everyday sense, to mean an upsetting condition in an individual occurring in response to adverse external influences, stressors. Stimulation of the aforementioned hypothalamic–pituitary–adrenal axis may lead to fleeting or prolonged tachycardia, hypertension, muscular tension, irritability, and depression.

Stress, as we define it, is aversive. We don't like it. We try to avoid it. Not only is it unpleasant, it may literally sicken us, perhaps through effects on the immune system (Sheps *et al.* 2002; Yang and Glaser 2002; Bunker *et al.* 2003; Joachim *et al.* 2003; Miller *et al.* 2004). Yet sometimes we may be unaware that we are under stress. Has a coworker, noticing evidence of stress in your demeanor, posture, or tone of voice, ever surprised you by asking if you were all right? Have you ever asked a coworker the same question? Sometimes we are just too preoccupied or busy to notice. Yet stress awareness is the first step to stress reduction.

The expression "one man's meat is another man's poison," applies to stressors. Nurse Steel may shrug off a patient's angry outburst whereas Nurse Straw may be shaken by it. We shall examine some character traits and coping mechanisms as relevant for dealing with stress.

Sources of nursing stress

Clearly different nursing practices encompass different stressors. Yet some stressors have been generally acknowledged for many years. A quarter century ago Gray-Toft and Anderson (1981) listed the following areas of occupational stressors for nurses: death and dying; conflict with physicians; being unprepared to deal with the emotional needs of patients and families; lack of support; conflict with other nurses and supervisors; workload; and uncertainty concerning treatment. The domains of these stressors are "work content, working conditions, social and labor relations, and conditions of employment" (Janssen *et al.* 1999).

A nurse reminisces:

> "I often think back over the years spanning my career; and for some reason, the course of the cholecystectomy frequently comes to mind. Not all that many years ago, the patient would arrive on the unit the afternoon before surgery with time to settle in, get to know the staff, and enjoy a good night's sleep. Recovery in the hospital took 10 to 14 days. Now patients awaken early in the morning, drive to our large medical center, struggle to finding a parking place, have their gallbladder removed, arrive in our unit post-operatively, and expect to be discharged that afternoon if laparoscopic surgery had been performed, or in one to three days otherwise. Is it any wonder that everyone feels the rush these days?"

Another nurse relates an interaction with an elderly gentleman who was ordered to drink a gallon of a potent laxative solution in two hours.

> "The more I urged him to drink up the quieter he became. The next morning this is what he told me: 'You were pushing me too much yesterday. I know my body better than you do, and I would have thrown up if I had taken it too fast.'
>
> I thanked him for his honesty. He added that he always explains how he feels and accepts how others feel, and if they can't agree, he walks away because life is just too short. His open and direct communication reminded me that time limits certainly exists – today more than ever – but that we remain in a *people* business."

The threat of violence as a stressor

There are, of course, other stressors. Some hospitals and perhaps especially their emergency departments (Fernandez *et al.* 1999) can be dangerous places compared with other occupational settings, but studies can vary widely in how they categorize violence, distinguish violence from abuse, survey the population, etc. A systematic literature search and critical review concluded that more than 9.5% of nurses in general U.K. hospitals could be expected to be assaulted, with or without injury, in one year (Wells and Bowers 2002). Twenty-seven percent of respondents in a recent study at one U.K. hospital (Winstanley and Whittington 2004) reported being assaulted in the previous year and of all the assaults nurses reported the most (43.4%) and doctors the least (13.8%). In the United States nurses may be three times more likely to experience workplace violence than other professionals (Keely 2002).

> "I was completely numb when that man pulled a knife on me. I didn't feel a thing but afterwards I had a long cry about it. And I had some dreams for a while, too."

During an eight month study in an American urban setting 3,446 metallic weapons, primarily knives and other cutting instruments, were confiscated from individuals entering the emergency room area of a general hospital compared with 260 from individuals entering the emergency room area of a children's hospital, both equipped with metal detectors. On average 500 weapons a month were confiscated from individuals at the two institutions (Simon *et al.* 2003). We experience stress simply reading the numbers.

Conflict

Poor relations with colleagues, even outright aggression among them, have been reported by nurses in various settings as a significant source of stress. Farrell (2001) discusses possible contributing factors, themselves stressful, including disenfranchising work practices, clique formation, poor self-esteem, nurse manager responses, intergenerational conflict, and others.

Swearingen and Liberman (2004) describe conflict between the Baby Boomer generation of nurses (born 1943–1960) and Generation X nurses (born 1960–1980) due to different values derived from entering the profession at different times.[2]

Conflict may be a source of stress but, engaged in constructively, can benefit the group by leading to better solutions to a problem than originally contemplated (Sessa 1998).

Involved in conflict with another person, a nurse will generally have two concerns: maintenance of the relationship and obtaining the goal. The relative value given to these concerns leads to different styles of conflict management: collaborative, compromising, accommodative, forcing, or avoidant (Bartol *et al.* 2001). Trust is best fostered between two individuals in conflict if a third party is not brought in to resolve it. Common sense steps to conflict management include the identification of the problem, expression of feelings, exploration of options, and evaluation of results (Antai-Otong 2001).

> "I used to immediately agree with whatever my supervisor said so I could just get away because she always made me nervous. But then after I left I was mad at myself. It would eat me up. I'm still nervous but now if I disagree I say so in a nice tone of voice and usually things work out and I'm not mad at myself anymore."[3]

Moral stress

When a nurse experiences empathic concern for a vulnerable patient, but is prevented because of external factors from doing what is best for the patient, the nurse experiences moral stress (Lutzen *et al.* 2003). These external factors may include high workload, lack of influence over work assignment, "limited avenues for skills development", and "diminishing support from supervisors" (Severinsson and Kamaker 1999; Henderson 2001; Sumner and Townsend-Rocchiccioli 2003).

Emotional contagion

Though emotional work was not always valued as such (Williams 2001), it is now widely understood as an inherent part of nursing care (Henderson 2001; Sumner and Townsend-Rocchiccioli 2003). Energy is required to work with people whose emotions are in turmoil. A person working at an airline ticket counter may need to expend some energy maintaining equanimity while dealing with passengers late for a departure. How much more emotional work must a nurse do in caring for a cancer patient terrified of a planned bone marrow aspiration or as in the following example trying to remain calm when being yelled at.

> Mr. Arrowwise, a gentleman in his late eighties, had undergone colon resection for a tumor and during his delirium had removed his IV line, nasogastric tube, urinary catheter, and other troubling appendages. He was more alert after narcotics were discontinued.
>
> As he and his wife walked the hall together, she stopped to ask me if I would please reassure him that he had hurt no one during his period of agitation. On hearing this he burst into an emotional description of his ongoing trial, including the banners hung all over the courtroom declaring his guilt.
>
> In my most professional and reassuring manner, I told Mr. Arrowwise that he had injured no one, that there was no trial, and that commonly people have bad dreams after surgery. He need not worry.
>
> Rather than calming him, my explanation infuriated him. His shouting drew everyone's attention. "You keep your nose out of this young lady and mind your own business . . . you know nothing about this. It is my trial and my courtroom and my physician will bring me the results. He will be here any minute!"
>
> I did not feel calm but in my calmest tone replied, "You know, Mr. Arrowwise, in that case, we will just wait for your physician to bring you the news." I left, cutting my losses. A peer who had witnessed this entire interaction caught my eye and, with a wink, mouthed the word "coward" for me to see. It made me laugh as he had intended. Being yelled at is painful.

One of the most interesting stressors potentially leading to burnout is emotional contagion,[4] the nurse's actual experience of the distressing emotions of a patient, literally feeling the anxiety of an anxious patient, the anger of an angry one, the grief of a grieving one, etc. Distinct from emotional contagion is empathy, the accurate perception and understanding of another's situation, feelings, and motives, which is generally regarded as an important part of caring for a patient. Omdahl and O'Donnell (1999) illustrate, however, how some nursing texts advocate empathic concern, "others insist on both concern and emotional contagion, and many leave the reader totally baffled as to whether one is or is not to share patients' emotions." Because emotional contagion but not empathy may contribute to burnout they recommend that nursing education teach nurses how to promote empathic concern but to avoid emotional contagion. To editorialize briefly, we concur, yet in some settings such contagion may be difficult to avoid (Kelly *et al.* 2002; Papadatou *et al.* 2002).

Burnout

Burnout for nurses is work-related emotional exhaustion. Patients become objects, or are generally found burdensome (de-personalization), and the nurse feels professionally ineffective. Energy cannot be summoned to work effectively (Maslach 1982). Theoretically any prolonged work-related stressor could lead to burnout.

Stress management

The role of nursing supervisors in reducing stress

Nurses face stress as the numbers of acutely ill patients increase along with "the pressure to conform to rigorous standards of cost-containment and quality assurance programmes" (Stordeur *et al.* 2001). Along with these changes nurses face the ever moving industrial conveyor belt delivering to them new computerized information systems,[5] infusion pumps, monitoring devices, medications, etc.

By remaining sensitive and supportive of staff, a head nurse "can buffer the effects of a demanding work environment. A tyrannical, excessively control-oriented head nurse, however, can increase staff stress – actually causing elevated systolic and diastolic blood pressures – with exhortations such as: 'work more quickly', 'work accurately', 'you could do more', 'hurry up, we haven't much time left'" (Stordeur *et al.* 2001).

Assertiveness and stress management techniques

Assertiveness among nurses is one approach to stress management (Antai-Otong 2001; Walczak and Absolon 2001; Buback 2004; Hertting *et al.* 2004). It takes some practice.

Relaxation and focusing techniques can help the individual and, of course, having a fulfilling life away from work is of enormous benefit, not only because of the respite of a happy home, but because one's self-confidence and stress tolerance are bolstered (Antai-Otong 2001).

An ancient technique of relaxation is controlled deep abdominal breathing. The inhalation is held for few seconds, followed by complete exhalation, a pause, and then another full inhalation. Find the rhythm that is completely comfortable. A time out from a stressful encounter, followed by this technique can save the day.

Though it is natural to ruminate over things that go wrong, an alternative approach is to resolve to do it differently next time. A nurse told us this story.

> "My brother-in-law Bob, a horse trainer, managed a grain elevator several years ago. When one of his employees failed to fill an order, an angry farmer appeared asking about his grain. Bob met with him, listened to his litany of complaints, then said, 'You will have your grain by Monday morning.' My sister was amazed. Why hadn't Bob explained to the farmer what had happened, why he wasn't to blame. 'Rose,' said Bob, 'all he is interested in is getting his grain. He will have it by Monday morning.' I have applied this to my career ever since. I do not tell patients that we are short of a nurse or a nurses' aid today – or whatever. This day is the patient's day, this time, the patient's time – to heal, to conquer, to endure. They should not have to hear why their grain wasn't ordered correctly; it is my job to see that they get it by Monday morning."

Concluding remarks

Many areas of nursing are stressful. Perhaps one of the articles listed in the reference section here will more specifically address the reader's concerns. We hope the reader will forgive us not citing popular books from the self-help literature. They are there for all to see.

Bibliography

Antai-Otong D. 2001 Creative stress-management techniques for self-renewal. *Dermatology Nursing*. 13(1):31–2, 35–9, Feb.

Atawneh FA. Zahid MA. Al-Sahlawi KS. Shahid AA. Al-Farrah MH. 2003 Violence against nurses in hospitals: prevalence and effects. *British Journal of Nursing*. 12(2):102–7, Jan 23–Feb 12.

Bailey M. Engler H. Hunzeker J. Sheridan JF. 2003 The hypothalamic–pituitary–adrenal axis and viral infection. *Viral Immunology*. 16(2):141–57.

Bartol GM. Parrish RS. McSweeney M. 2001 Effective conflict management begins with knowing your style. *Journal for Nurses in Staff Development*. 17(1):34–40, Jan–Feb.

Buback D. 2004 Assertiveness training to prevent verbal abuse in the OR. *AORN Journal*. 79(1):148–50, 153–8, 161–4: quiz 165–6, 169–70, Jan.

Bunker SJ. Colquhoun DM. Esler MD. Hickie IB. Hunt D. Jelinek VM. Oldenburg BF. Peach HG. Ruth D. Tennant CC. Tonkin AM. 2003 "Stress" and coronary heart disease: psychosocial risk factors. *Medical Journal of Australia*. 178(6):272–6, Mar 17.

Buxman K. 2000 Humor in critical care: no joke. *AACN Clinical Issues*. 11(1):120–7, Feb.

Clum GA. Luscomb RL. Scott L. 1982 Relaxation training and cognitive redirection strategies in the treatment of acute pain. *Pain*. 12:175.

Currell R. Urquhart C. 2003 Nursing record systems: effects on nursing practice and health care outcomes. [update of *Cochrane Database Syst Rev*. 2000;(2):CD002099; PMID: 10796679]. *Cochrane Database of Systematic Reviews*. (3):CD002099.

Davidhizar R. Eshleman J. Wolff LA. 2001 Coping with a heightened level of stress. *Journal of Practical Nursing*. 51(4):12–15; quiz 16–7, Winter.

De Bellis A. Longson D. Glover P. Hutton A. 2001 The enculturation of our nursing graduates. *Contemporary Nurse*. 11(1):84–94, Sep.

Edwards D. Burnard P. A systematic review of stress and stress management interventions for mental health nurses. *Journal of Advanced Nursing*. 42(2):169–200, Apr.

Farrell GA. 2001 From tall poppies to squashed weeds*: why don't nurses pull together more? *Journal of Advanced Nursing*. 35(1):26–33, Jul.

Fernandez CM. Bouthillette F. Rabbound JM, *et al*. 1999 Violence in the emergency department: a survey of health care workers. *Canadian Medical Association Journal*. 161 (10):1245–48.

Froggatt K. 1998 The place of metaphor and language in exploring nurses' emotional work. *Journal of Advanced Nursing*. 28(2):332–8, Aug.

Gray-Toft P. Anderson JG. 1981 The nursing stress scale; development of an instrument. *Journal of Behavioral Assessment* 3:11–23.

Haddad JJ. Saade NE. Safieh-Garabedian B. 2002 Cytokines and neuro-immune-endocrine interactions: a role for the hypothalamic–pituitary–adrenal revolving axis. [erratum appears in *J Neuroimmunol*. 2003 Dec;145(1–2):154]. *Journal of Neuroimmunology*. 133(1–2):1–19, Dec.

Healy CM. McKay MF. 2000 Nursing stress: the effects of coping strategies and job satisfaction in a sample of Australian nurses. [erratum appears in *J Adv Nurs* 2000 Apr;31(4):989]. *Journal of Advanced Nursing*. 31(3):681–8, Mar.

Henderson A. 2001 Emotional labor and nursing: an under-appreciated aspect of caring work. *Nursing Inquiry*. 8(2):130–8, Jun.

Hertting A. Nilsson K. Theorell T. Larsson US. 2004 Downsizing and reorganization: demands, challenges and ambiguity for registered nurses. *Journal of Advanced Nursing*. 45(2):145–54, Jan.

Herzog AC. 2000 Conflict resolution in a nutshell: tips for everyday nursing. *SCI Nursing*. 17(4):162–6, Winter.

Heuser I. Lammers CH. 2003 Stress and the brain. *Neurobiology of Aging*. 24 (Suppl 1):S69–76; discussion S81–2, May–Jun.

Janssen PPM. de Jonge J. Bakker AB. 1999 Specific determinants of intrinsic work motivation, burnout and turnover intentions: a study among nurses. *Journal of Advanced Nursing.* 29:1360–9.

Joachim RA. Quarcoo D. Arck PC. Herz U. Renz H. Klapp BF. 2003 Stress enhances airway reactivity and airway inflammation in an animal model of allergic bronchial asthma. *Psychosomatic Medicine.* 65(5):811–5, Sep–Oct.

Keely BR. 2002 Recognition and prevention of hospital violence. *Dimensions of Critical Care Nursing.* 21(6):236–41, Nov–Dec.

Kelly D. Ross S. Gray B. Smith P. 2002 Death, dying and emotional labour: problematic dimensions of the bone marrow transplant nursing role? *Journal of Advanced Nursing.* 32(4):952–60, Oct.

Lutzen K. Cronqvist A. Magnusson A. Andersson L. 2003 Moral stress: synthesis of a concept. *Nursing Ethics: an International Journal for Health Care Professionals.* 10(3):312–22, May.

Marino PA. 1998 The effects of cumulative grief in the nurse. *Journal of Intravenous Nursing.* 21(2):101–4, Mar–Apr.

Maslach C. 1982 *Burnout: the Cost of Caring.* Englewood Cliffs, N.J.: Prentice Hall.

McVicar A. 2003 Workplace stress in nursing: a literature review. *Journal of Advanced Nursing.* 44(6):633–42, Dec.

Miller GE. Cohen S. Pressman S. Barkin A. Rabin BS. Treanor JJ. 2004 Psychological stress and antibody response to influenza vaccination: when is the critical period for stress, and how does it get inside the body? *Psychosomatic Medicine.* 66(2):215–23.

Omdahl BL. O'Donnell C. 1999 Emotional contagion, empathic concern and communicative responsiveness as variables affecting nurses' stress and occupational commitment. *Journal of Advanced Nursing.* 29(6):1351–9, Jun.

Papadatou D. Bellali T. Papazoglou I. Petraki D. 2002 Greek nurse and physician grief as a result of caring for children dying of cancer. *Pediatric Nursing.* 28(4):345–53, Jul–Aug.

Payne N. 2001 Occupational stressors and coping as determinants of burnout in female hospice nurses. *Journal of Advanced Nursing.* 33(3):396–405, Feb.

Peteet JR. Evans KR. 1991 Problematic behavior of drug-dependent patients in the general hospital. A clinical and administrative approach to management. *General Hospital Psychiatry.* 13(3):150–5, May.

Rushen J. 1986 Some problems with the physiological concept of "stress". *Australian Veterinary Journal.* 63(11):359–61, Nov.

Santamaria N. 2000 The relationship between nurses' personality and stress levels reported when caring for interpersonally difficult patients. *Australian Journal of Advanced Nursing.* 18(2):20–6, Dec–Feb.

Selye H. 1985 The nature of stress. *Basal Facts.* 7(1):3–11.

Sessa VI. 1998 Using conflict to improve effectiveness of nurse teams. *Orthopaedic Nursing.* 17(3):41–6; quiz 47–8, May–Jun.

Severinsson EI. Kamaker D. 1999 Clinical nursing supervision in the workplace – effects on moral stress and job satisfaction. *Journal of Nursing Management.* 7(2):81–90, Mar.

Sheps DS. McMahon RP. Becker L, *et al.* 2002 Mental-stress induced ischemia and all-cause mortality in patients with coronary heart disease. *Circulation.* 105:1780–4.

Simon HK. Khan NS. Delgado CA. 2003 Weapons detection at two urban hospitals. *Pediatric Emergency Care.* 19(4):248–51, Aug.

Stordeur S. D'hoore W. Vandenberghe C. 2001 Leadership, organizational stress, and emotional exhaustion among hospital nursing staff. *Journal of Advanced Nursing.* 35(4):533–42, Aug.

Sumner J. Townsend-Rocchiccioli J. 2003 Why are nurses leaving nursing?. *Nursing Administration Quarterly.* 27(2):164–71, Apr–Jun.

Swearingen S. Liberman A. 2004 Nursing generations: an expanded look at the emergence of conflict and its resolution. *Health Care Manager.* 23(1):54–64, Jan–Mar.

van Londen L. Hes JP. Ameling EH. Hengeveld MW. 1990 Staff attitudes toward violence in the general hospital. A comparison between Amsterdam and Tel Aviv. *General Hospital Psychiatry*. 12(4):252–6, Jul.

Walczak MB. Absolon PL. 2001 Essentials for effective communication in oncology nursing: assertiveness, conflict management, delegation, and motivation. [republished in *J Nurses Staff Dev*. 2001 May–Jun;17(3):159–62; PMID: 11998676]. *Journal for Nurses in Staff Development* 17(2):67–70, Mar–Apr.

Wells J. Bowers L. 2002 How prevalent is violence towards nurses working in general hospitals in the UK?. *Journal of Advanced Nursing*. 39(3):230–40, Aug.

Williams A. 2001 A literature review on the concept of intimacy in nursing. *Journal of Advanced Nursing*. 33(5):660–7, Mar.

Winstanley S. Whittington R. 2004 Aggression towards health care staff in a UK general hospital: variation among professions and departments. *Journal of Clinical Nursing*. 13(1):3–10, Jan.

Yang EV. Glaser R. 2002 Stress-induced immunomodulation and the implications for health. *International Immunopharmacology*. 2(2–3):315–24, Feb.

Chapter 13

Getting psychiatric consultation

We begin by discussing the terms consultation, referral, and liaison. For a nurse or physician to ask for psychiatric *consultation*, is to ask a psychiatric nurse or psychiatrist to review a case, examine the patient, and make recommendations regarding diagnosis and treatment. To *refer* a patient to a psychiatric nurse or psychiatrist is to ask the specialist to provide care for the patient. A *liaison* psychiatric nurse or psychiatrist is one who is a regular member of the treatment team, not one who is called only for consultation, or referred to from time to time. A *consultation/liaison* psychiatric nurse or psychiatrist[1] does provide consultation but is also routinely present and available on the ward as a member of the treatment team.

Although having a psychiatric consultant available in the setting of a general hospital is widely seen as valuable[2] (Alaja *et al.* 1999; Chadda 2001; Rigatelli *et al.* 2001; Sharrock and Happell 2002a, b), availability of services varies greatly from hospital-to-hospital, city-to-city, and country-to-country, as do the arrangements by which these services are paid for. If psychiatric consultation/liaison services are available they will be used. The joke among physicians is that success as a consultant depends on three A's in decreasing order of importance: availability, affability, and ability. There is some backing in the literature for this notion (Langley and Till 1989).

There are, of course, psychiatrists in most major cities, some of them available for referral or consultation. Most helpful in the hospital are those consultants specially trained and interested in consultation/liaison psychiatry, the branch of psychiatry addressing the psychosocial aspects of medical care. These specialists work closely with the medical, nursing, and other staff in the management of patients whose primary diagnosis is non-psychiatric.

Consultation versus consultation/liaison

As noted, a request for consultation generally means a request for advice. In our hospital, a tertiary referral center, what physicians really want is a consultant who will not simply give advice, but also take over the psychiatric aspects of their patient's care, see the patient regularly, and help the house staff and nursing staff caring for the patient. Physicians are dissatisfied if the consultant, for example, makes a diagnosis and recommends a treatment or approach, but does not follow the patient regularly to make adjustments. Generally these patients are difficult, with complex problems, and they tend to have longer than average hospital stays.

A consultation-liaison psychiatrist on staff gets to know the other physicians well, a great advantage in providing help tailored to the individual physician requesting help with a difficult patient. Trust between physicians can lead to swift resolution of problems as this case history illustrates:

> The nurse on an orthopedic unit asked the orthopedic surgeon for a psychiatric consultation to help with the care of Ms. J. C. a 54-year-old woman with a complex medical and psychiatric history. She suffered from diabetes mellitus, and chronic abdominal pain for which she had received oral narcotics for years. She had undergone a knee replacement because of degenerative joint disease but the prosthesis had become infected and she was admitted for its removal. It was temporarily replaced with a cement block impregnated with antibiotics. Most patients would have been sitting by day one and bearing weight by day two, but Ms. J.C. screamed if her leg were moved, forbade the nurse from changing dressings or even moving the sheets at times.
>
> On day three the physical therapist called the consultation/liaison psychiatrist who until this time had focused on the patient's depression and pain management. It was immediately clear to him that no amount of negotiation would work. Muscle spasm and pain were expected after this procedure but what the patient reported was far out of proportion to physical findings or expectations. The consultation/ liaison psychiatrist, who knew the orthopedic surgeon well, arranged a meeting in the patient's room the next day to include the surgeon, the physician's assistant, the physical therapist, the nurse, the medical social worker, the medical resident, and the patient's friend.
>
> The orthopedic surgeon stood at the bedside and asked why it was so hard to move. The patient said the pain was intolerable. The surgeon said that pain was expected, that he'd performed similar procedures on hundreds of patients who by this time were standing. In a gentle, professional manner he told her she had no choice. The psychiatrist suggested to the patient that with everyone present she should be moved up in the bed. She said no. The orthopedic surgeon again said she had no choice. The surgeon braced her leg while the physical therapist and the physician's assistant moved her toward the head of the bed. She cried out and began sobbing. While still sobbing, she was asked by the surgeon what was so bad about that. The pain, she said. But she had stopped crying. The psychiatrist asked the physical therapist, who had called him in the first place, what else would help. Getting the patient to the side of the bed now, said the therapist. They proceeded to do so, again with another bout of loud crying. Then the patient was moved to the commode. That afternoon the patient was fully engageable, not crying. She maintained her greatly increased mobility, permitted nurses and therapist to care for her, and was discharged to a nursing home two days later.

Note that the physical therapist could not have proceeded against the patient's wishes without the backing of the orthopedic surgeon. Furthermore even the experienced orthopedic physician's assistant, the surgical resident, and the nurse worried about doing some harm given the patient's dramatic behavior. The psychiatrist was not about to insist that the patient move either. Only the orthopedic surgeon, who had performed the operation, fully understood the anatomy and physiology of the patient's condition had no fear of doing harm. He calmly helped the physical therapist do what needed to be done.

Everyone involved in the patient's care, including the patient's companion, was present to see and hear for themselves what moving the patient entailed.

The psychiatrist's role was to understand that neither negotiation nor more aggressive use of narcotics would make any difference. He was on a first name basis with the surgeon and communication between them was quick and easy.

This case illustrates how the attending physician's support of staff is absolutely necessary in certain cases, how limit setting must be done by physicians as well as nurses, and how the psychiatric consultant may be effective simply by mobilizing the team to communicate among themselves and set limits. This is liaison work.

Attitudes of nurses and doctors towards psychiatric consultation

General hospital nurses often lack confidence in their ability to care for patients with psychiatric problems and are grateful for help. In the med/surg setting a psychiatric consultation/liaison nurse can educate nurses in the care of these patients (Sharrock and Happell 2002a, b). Such an arrangement might even shorten length of hospital stay (de Jonge et al. 2003), though studies demonstrating this are difficult and rare, in part because great variance in length of stay makes necessary very large studies to show a difference between experimental groups (patients who had the benefit of psychiatric consultation) and control groups (Andreoli et al. 2003).

Perhaps because they are concerned that patients will feel stigmatized, physicians in some settings may be reluctant to involve a psychiatrist in the care of their patients (Koran et al. 1979; Swigar et al. 1992; Chadda 2001; Smaira et al. 2003). We believe that hospital nurses, because they are with their troubled patients all day long, are generally more attuned to the need for psychiatric care in their patients (Pasacreta and Massie 1990; Shahinpour et al. 1995; Kurlowicz 2001; Sharrock and Happell 2002b).

Although some physicians are reluctant to obtain psychiatric consultation, we believe many more are frustrated by the lack of psychiatric consultants dedicated to helping care for their medical patients (Ito et al. 1999). The literature suggests that once consultation is obtained, however, both patients and physicians more often find it helpful than not (Koran et al. 1979; Windgassen et al. 1997; Rigatelli. et al. 2001).

For certain patient populations much psychiatric morbidity goes unrecognized and untreated (Chadda 2001; Fallowfield et al. 2001; Torres-Harding et al. 2002; Lowe et al. 2003; Walker et al. 2003; Shores et al. 2004). More frequent use of psychiatric consultants can sensitize treating physicians and nurses.

Precipitants of psychiatric consultation

If a consultation/liaison nurse is on the hospital staff, another nurse may simply ask the first to evaluate the patient and make recommendations to the team. In some settings it is necessary for a physician to ask for psychiatric consultation, but even in these cases it is probably the nurse who has identified a problem in the first place. Nurses are attuned to the distress of their patients. We now comment on some areas, already discussed elsewhere, that warrant consideration of psychiatric consultation.

Substance abuse or dependence, including alcohol

In one study on the medical and surgical wards of a general hospital the introduction of a specialist, an addictions trained psychiatric nurse, led to 88% completion of alcohol rehabilitation of those patients entering treatment compared with the previous 40% completion rate with the traditional assessment service, which did include psychiatric consultants who, however, did not have specialist training (Hillman *et al.* 2001). Other programs also report encouraging results of psychiatric consultation regarding alcohol or other substance abuse (Alaja and Seppa 2003). Alcohol-related disorders in some settings are the primary diagnoses in patients for whom psychiatric consultation is requested (Smaira *et al.* 2003).

Unfortunately even when hospital admission blood alcohol levels are 300 mg/deciliter or above, an "unsubtle" level, alcohol-related disorders are not assessed, particularly on trauma units (Bostwick and Seaman 2004).

> Mrs. P, 40, a homemaker has been admitted to the hospital for the third time for unexplained falls at home. Psychiatric consultation is requested. The patient is pleasant, vague, and slow. Her short-term memory is slightly impaired. Sitting at the bedside the psychiatrist asks if he may, in her presence, go through her purse to see what medications she may have forgotten to mention. The psychiatrist discovers five bottles of various tranquilizers, and several loose pills, which he has the pharmacy identify. In the context of marital discord, she has been taking large doses of tranquilizers. He speaks with her physicians and with her husband and daughter. The patient is confronted and accepts referral to a chemical dependency specialist. The patient no longer falls at home.

The patient who demands narcotics

When patients ask that their intravenous narcotic or diphenhydramine be administered quickly – "Give it to me fast!" – experienced nurses may see a red flag, a warning that drug seeking may be motivated more by a desire for escape than for relief of physical pain.

> Jim C. was admitted from St. Elsewhere with necrotizing gallstone pancreatitis. A self-described hard working type-A personality, he had ignored his family physician's recommendation that he undergo cholecystectomy after evaluation of his right upper quadrant pain revealed a gallbladder filled with stones. He drove a truck 16 hours a day to support his large family. He had a machine shop in his garage.
>
> Mr. C. was extremely anxious, requiring much support for every procedure. Progress was slow as it often is with this syndrome. With time, however, he became more relaxed and trusting. He did, however, continue to request intravenous hydromorphone even after he began eating and taking other medications by mouth. His primary nurse became alarmed when he began saying "Give it fast so I can feel the rush in my head and know that I've had it."
>
> Aware that the hydromorphone contributed to his severe constipation he decided one morning to stop asking for it. By midafternoon he was anxious and tearful, but not because of pain. He simply felt "out of control". His nurse asked for

psychiatric consultation, which then revealed the primacy of the patient's anxiety and depression. He had been masking with hydromorphone. The psychiatrist ordered clonazepam 0.25 mg by mouth every 12 hours which immediately reduced his anxiety, fluoxetine for both anxiety and depression, and methadone 5 mg by mouth for pain on a prn basis.[3]

The results were dramatic. In the next 24 hours, Jim requested the methadone only once and was grateful for the decrease in his anxiety. The psychiatrist came by daily for a while. Mr. C's complaint of pain almost disappeared.

Almost every experienced hospital nurse has seen similar scenarios deteriorate into incessant and inappropriate demands for narcotics, not for the soma but for the psyche, to numb the emotional pain of depression, anxiety, or boredom. None of us wish to see our patients suffer but often narcotics are not the answer. The psychiatric consultant can sort out the underlying problems and outline a treatment plan.

Lucy J, 25, living with her grandmother, was repeatedly admitted to the hospital with presumed diabetic gastropathy, abdominal pain, and nausea. She had failed to care for herself, failed to attend scheduled appointments, and failed to use narcotics in the manner prescribed. Despite this history the gastroenterologist agreed to provide her with a gastric pacemaker if she promised to reform her ways. After the operation, however, Ms. J refused insulin, refused to get out of bed, refused to shower or attend to personal hygiene even when repeatedly offered assistance. She demanded frequent doses of hydromorphone, screaming and cursing when higher doses were denied. Once she got out of bed, walked to the nurses' station, and sat on the floor, refusing to move unless her hydromorphone dose was increased.

Her grandmother was incensed at what she perceived to be poor nursing care, for Ms. J had told her that no one would help her out of bed and that she hadn't showered or received any personal care in three days.

Psychiatric consultation and a team conference were arranged. A plan of care was determined and presented to Ms. J by her physician, nurse, and psychiatric consultant. That night Ms. J. cut her forearms superficially with scissors. She refused to speak with the psychiatrist who then called the county designated mental health professional (CDMHP)[4] to evaluate her for involuntary commitment. Ms. J. disclosed to the CDMHP that she had not attempted suicide but rather tried to get attention and receive more intravenous hydromorphone. After spending two hours with her, he told her he thought her pain was more psychological than physical. Ms. J. then called her grandmother relating a warped version of the meeting. An hour later Ms. J's grandmother berated the nurse by phone for not giving her granddaughter more IV hydromophone, as she understood the CDMHP to have recommended. The consultation/liaison psychiatrist met with Ms. J and her grandmother to review the entire situation including what the CDMHP had actually said. When Ms. J realized that the plan of care and the dose of hydromorphone were unchanged she demanded immediate discharge.

Although Ms. J. remained manipulative throughout her hospitalization, limits were adhered to. Despite her provocations, she and her grandmother were always treated respectfully, addressed politely, and given the time – considerable time – to express their distress. Without psychiatric consultation Ms. J would have been hospitalized for much longer, exposing her to the dangers of over-sedation, blood clots, falls, infection, etc. Most patients are discharged within 24 hours after gastric pacemaker placement.

Older patients with cognitive or emotional disturbance

Older patients with cognitive disorders, substance abuse, depression, and other problems are referred for psychiatric consultation much less frequently than would be useful. In one study only 3% of older patients with retrospectively identified problems received consultations (Swigar *et al.* 1992). Eighty-eight percent of old age psychiatrists[5] in one survey were unhappy with the consultation model, which required the identification of a problem before asking for consultation. They thought that older people and staff would best be served by a liaison model of service (Holmes *et al.* 2003). Involvement of a psychiatric consultation/liaison nurse, for example, may not only improve the care of older people but, as noted earlier, help educate nurses in the care of these patients (Kurlowicz 2001).

> Mrs. Beardsley, 86, has just undergone hip surgery but insists that she must leave the hospital now because of things she has to do at home. She's fully oriented and alert but it is difficult to understand the urgency of her request. The consultation/ liaison psychiatrist is asked to see her. He speaks with her gently, eventually getting around to ask if she feels safe in the hospital. "Would you feel safe if someone were trying to kill you?"
> The patient has become delusional post-operatively.[6] The psychiatrist orders a dose of an antipsychotic medication, the patient's anxiety subsides, and she agrees to stay in hospital for a day or two longer.

Depression and suicide

Patients who commit suicide while in a general hospital or soon after being discharged from one suffer from major depression and other mental disorders, including substance abuse, just as do people who commit suicide outside the general hospital setting (Suominen *et al.* 2002). Current or recent general hospital patients are probably at much higher risk for suicide than those not recently hospitalized. The incidence of suicide after general hospital discharge in one study was three times higher than in the general population, but only one patient of 11 suicides and 33 controls had been referred for consultation (Dhossche *et al.* 2001). In another study, internists and surgeons recognized as depressed only about a third of the depressed patients under their care (Balestrieri *et al.* 2002).

> Mr. D, 64, an abstinent alcoholic with lung cancer is in the hospital for pneumonia. He keeps the shades drawn, is laconic and gruff, and has no visitors. His nurse is uneasy caring for him and asks the attending physician if perhaps a psychiatrist should be called. The doctor concurs. When the psychiatrist asks directly about

suicide and the possible means to complete it, the patient points to a bag full of sleeping pills.

Trauma patients

Patients who have suffered burns may have a broad range of issues for which psychiatric consultation is needed (Ilechukwu 2002). Trauma patients may go for years before their psychiatric difficulties, including post-traumatic stress disorder, are diagnosed (Davis and Breslau 1994).

Angry patients

As noted elsewhere ignoring anger paradoxically may increase it and the threat of violence by worsening distrust, paranoia, and feelings of helplessness (Atkinson 1982; Morrison *et al*. 2000). If the nurses on staff are unable to manage the anger themselves (Thomas 1998), consultation may be advisable.

Concluding remarks

In 1998 a major medical center in Seattle announced that, because of fiscal constraints, it was terminating the employment of the consultation/liaison psychiatrist who for years had helped manage difficult patients on the medical and surgical wards of its general hospital. Within a few days of the announcement a surgeon and gastro-enterologist circulated a petition signed by hundreds of nurses, physicians, physical therapists, ward clerks, and others requesting that the administration reconsider its decision, which it promptly did.

Bibliography

Alaja R. Seppa K. 2003 Six-month outcomes of hospital-based psychiatric substance use consultations. *General Hospital Psychiatry*. 25(2):103–7, Mar–Apr.

Alaja R. Tienari P. Seppa K. Tuomisto M. Leppavuori A. Huyse FJ. Herzog T. Malt UF. Lobo A. 1999 Patterns of comorbidity in relation to functioning (GAF) among general hospital psychiatric referrals. European Consultation-Liaison Workgroup. *Acta Psychiatrica Scandinavica*. 99(2):135–40, Feb.

Andreoli PB. Citero Vde A. Mari Jde J. 2003 A systematic review of studies of the cost-effectiveness of mental health consultation-liaison interventions in general hospitals. *Psychosomatics*. 44(6):499–507, Nov–Dec.

Atkinson JH Jr. 1982 Managing the violent patient in the general hospital. *Postgraduate Medicine*. 71(1):193–7, 200–1, Jan.

Balestrieri M. Bisoffi G. Tansella M. Martucci M. Goldberg DP. 2002 Identification of depression by medical and surgical general hospital physicians. *General Hospital Psychiatry*. 24(1):4–11, Jan–Feb.

Bostwick JM. Seaman JS. 2004 Hospitalized patients and alcohol: who is being missed?. *General Hospital Psychiatry*. 26(1):59–62, Jan–Feb.

Brown JB. Weston WW. 1992 A survey of residency-trained family physicians and their referral of psychosocial problems. *Family Medicine*. 24(3):193–6, Mar–Apr.

Chadda RK. 2001 Psychiatry in non-psychiatric setting – a comparative study of physicians and surgeons. *Journal of the Indian Medical Association*. 99(1):24, 26–7, 62, Jan.

Chase P. Gage J. Stanley KM. Bonadonna JR. 2000 The psychiatric consultation/liaison nurse role in case management. *Nursing Case Management*. 5(2):73–7, Mar–Apr.

Davis GC. Breslau N. 1994 Post-traumatic stress disorder in victims of civilian trauma and criminal violence. *Psychiatric Clinics of North America*. 17(2):289–99, Jun.

de Jonge P. Latour CH. Huyse FJ. 2003 Implementing psychiatric interventions on a medical ward: effects on patients' quality of life and length of hospital stay. *Psychosomatic Medicine*. 65(6):997–1002, Nov–Dec.

Dhossche DM. Ulusarac A. Syed W. 2001 A retrospective study of general hospital patients who commit suicide shortly after being discharged from the hospital. *Archives of Internal Medicine*. 161(7):991–4, Apr 9.

Fallowfield L. Ratcliffe D. Jenkins V. Saul J. 2001 Psychiatric morbidity and its recognition by doctors in patients with cancer. *British Journal of Cancer*. 84(8):1011–15, Apr 20.

Gilbody SM. House AO. Sheldon TA. 2001 Routinely administered questionnaires for depression and anxiety: systematic review. *British Medical Journal*. 322(7283):406–9, Feb 17.

Hillman A. McCann B. Walker NP. 2001 Specialist alcohol liaison services in general hospitals improve engagement in alcohol rehabilitation and treatment outcome. *Health Bulletin*. 59(6):420–3, Nov.

Holmes J. Bentley K. Cameron I. 2003 A UK survey of psychiatric services for older people in general hospitals. *International Journal of Geriatric Psychiatry*. 18(8):716–21, Aug.

Ilechukwu ST. 2002 Psychiatry of the medically ill in the burn unit. *Psychiatric Clinics of North America*. 25(1):129–47, Mar.

Ito H. Kishi Y. Kurosawa H. 1999 A preliminary study of staff perception of psychiatric services in general hospitals. *General Hospital Psychiatry*. 21(1):57–61, Jan–Feb.

Jones A. 1997 Family therapy in a critical care unit. *Nursing Standard*. 11(21):40–2, Feb 12.

Koran LM. Van Natta J. Stephens JR. Pascualy R. 1979 Patients' reactions to psychiatric consultation. *Journal of the American Medical Association*. 241(15):1603–5, Apr 13.

Kurlowicz LH. 2001 Benefits of psychiatric consultation-liaison nurse interventions for older hospitalized patients and their nurses. *Archives of Psychiatric Nursing*. 15(2):53–61, Apr.

Langley GR. Till JE. 1989 Exemplary family physicians and consultants: empirical definition of contemporary medical practice. *Canadian Medical Association Journal*. 141(4):301–7, Aug 15.

Lowe B. Grafe K. Kroenke K. Zipfel S. Quenter A. Wild B. Fiehn C. Herzog W. 2003 Predictors of psychiatric comorbidity in medical outpatients. *Psychosomatic Medicine*. 65(5):764–70, Sep–Oct.

Morrison EF. Ramsey A. Synder BA. 2000 Managing the care of complex, difficult patients in the medical-surgical setting. *MEDSURG Nursing*. 9(1):21–6, Feb.

Pasacreta JV. Massie MJ. 1990 Nurses' reports of psychiatric complications in patients with cancer. *Oncology Nursing Forum*. 17(3):347–53, May–Jun.

Petrie K. 1989 Recent general practice contacts of hospitalised suicide attempters. *New Zealand Medical Journal*. 102(864):130–1, Mar 22.

Rigatelli M. Casolari L. Massari I. Ferrari S. 2001 A follow-up study of psychiatric consultations in the general hospital: What happens to patients after discharge?. *Psychotherapy & Psychosomatics*. 70(5):276–82, Sep–Oct.

Shahinpour N. Hollinger-Smith L. Perlia MA. 1995 The medical-psychiatric consultation liaison nurse. Meeting psychosocial needs of medical patients in the acute care setting. *Nursing Clinics of North America*. 30(1):77–86, Mar.

Sharrock J. Happell B. 2002a The psychiatric consultation-liaison nurse: thriving in a general hospital setting. *International Journal of Mental Health Nursing*. 11(1):24–33, Mar.

Sharrock J. Happell B. 2002b The role of a psychiatric consultation liaison nurse in a general hospital: a case study approach. *Australian Journal of Advanced Nursing*. 20(1):39–44, Sep–Nov.

Shores MM. Ryan-Dykes P. Williams RM. Mamerto B. Sadak T. Pascualy M. Felker BL. Zweigle M. Nichol P. Peskind ER. 2004 Identifying undiagnosed dementia in residential care veterans: comparing telemedicine to in-person clinical examination. *International Journal of Geriatric Psychiatry*. 19(2):101–8, Feb.

Smaira SI. Kerr-Correa F. Contel JO. 2003 Psychiatric disorders and psychiatric consultation in a general hospital: a case-control study. *Revista Brasileira de Psiquiatria*. 25(1):18–25, Mar.

Suominen K. Isometsa E. Heila H. Lonnqvist J. Henriksson M. 2002 General hospital suicides – a psychological autopsy study in Finland. *General Hospital Psychiatry*. 24(6):412–16, Nov–Dec.

Swigar ME. Sanguineti VR. Piscatelli RL. 1992 A retrospective study on the perceived need for and actual use of psychiatric consultations in older medical patients. *International Journal of Psychiatry in Medicine*. 22(3):239–49.

Thomas SP. 1998 Assessing and intervening with anger disorders. *Nursing Clinics of North America*. 33(1):121–33, Mar.

Torres-Harding SR. Jason LA. Cane V. Carrico A. Taylor RR. 2002 Physicians' diagnoses of psychiatric disorders for people with chronic fatigue syndrome. *International Journal of Psychiatry in Medicine*. 32(2):109–24.

Walker EA. Katon W. Russo J. Ciechanowski P. Newman E. Wagner AW. 2003 Health care costs associated with posttraumatic stress disorder symptoms in women. *Archives of General Psychiatry*. 60(4):369–74, Apr.

Windgassen K. Weissen PH. Schmidt K. 1997 [Prejudice and judgment: psychiatric consultation from the viewpoint of the patient]. [German] *Psychiatrische Praxis*. 24(3):134–7, May.

Zarr ML. 1991 Patient dynamics, staff burnout, and consultation-liaison psychiatry. *Physician Executive*. 17(5):37–40, Sep–Oct.

Notes

1 Mental status assessment

1   Did you know that six or more café au lait spots may be pathognomonic for neurofibromatosis, von Recklinghausen's disease?

2   This word, derived from the Greek, literally means not sitting down, or unable to sit still. It refers to a disturbing crawling sensation deep in the muscles, which the patient tries to relieve by moving about. In the hospital setting it is often caused by phenothiazines such as prochlorperazine (Compazine). Prochlorperazine may cause an acute dystonia as well.

2 Substance abuse

1   Here a substance refers to a drug of abuse, a medication, or a toxin and includes alcohol, amphetamines, cannabis, cocaine, hallucinogens, inhalants, nicotine, opioids, phencyclidine, sedatives, hypnotics, and anxiolytics (Bailes 1998). We may use the words substance and drug interchangeably.

2   A maladaptive pattern of use in the hospital, even if not lasting for twelve months, will still be referred to as abuse, though it would not meet strict diagnostic criteria.

3   This list is taken almost verbatim from the DSM IV.

4   The syndrome of withdrawal is different for different substances. See, for example, the table on narcotic withdrawal.

5   Actually amphetamines are sometimes ordered as appropriate stimulants and cocaine may be used in Brompton's cocktail (Davis 1978).

6   The term "addicted" has fallen out of favor, presumably because it is viewed as derogatory, but its meaning is clearer than the term "chemically dependent" since a person can be physiologically dependent on opioids but not addicted, i.e., the patient would experience a narcotic withdrawal syndrome were the administration of narcotics to cease, but obtaining and using narcotics is not the primary motivating factor in the patient's day-to-day life.

7   Six hours between doses of oral analgesics may still have its place as the total 24 hour dose of opioid is tapered and what is being treated is not so much pain as it is opioid dependence.

3 Delirium

1   Dr. Manos has personally treated over a thousand agitated delirious patients with IV haloperidol and only seen one case of it.

4 Psychiatric diagnoses

1   Note that the intern was later dismissed from the residency program for reasons presumably related to poor judgment, not based on this case alone.

5 Setting limits

1   One is tempted to say, "For crying out loud, behave yourself!"
2   Others may wish to attend such as physical therapists, medical social workers, and family members.
3   Do not speak of discharge if the physician in charge is not willing or able to discharge the patient for breaking of the agreement.

6 The nurse's authority

1   In the event of discharge, the physician would likely set up an outpatient follow-up appointment.
2   If you are the only person on the staff having difficulty with Mr. Mellacreesent you may wish to ask yourself privately if he reminds you of some important figure in your past whom you hated. If you are the only person on the staff who likes working with Mr. Mellacreesent you may wish to ask yourself if he reminds you of some important figure in your past whom you loved. Reacting to someone as if they were someone else is called countertransference. Sometimes awareness of countertransference helps us put our feelings in perspective. We raise the question for your interest.

8 The ethics of limit setting

1   In a sense the person is not himself.
2   All right, the nurse doesn't really recall this.
3   She might well be able to make rational decisions about other matters.

9 Families

1   Though it is "old" bones, "old" hearts, and "old" brains that cause our patients problems, in industrial societies "senior" has replaced "old" as an adjective for people of age greater than 65 because "old" is viewed as derogatory. Euphemisms hinder understanding but diplomacy may demand them.
2   Hedwig the owl in the Harry Potter movies might be a celebrity in a veterinary hospital if it weren't a primarily digital construction.

10 Communicating with doctors – the difficult and the easy

1   Most nurses then as now were women, a foundation of the game.
2   See, we said it again.
3   Because it is unsanitary and because it will lose its flavor.
4   When asked what his training for such meetings was this pulmonologist said his wife was a nurse.
5   During the holiday season a nurse at our hospital gave each of her colleagues a silk fortune cookie containing the message, "There will be harmony in the work place."

11 The nurse and the dying patient

1   Death anxiety does not refer to anticipatory grief and anxiety about the imminent death of a friend, relative, or self. It is a more long lasting state of mind.
2   Uncontrolled pain may be worse than death (Kulbe 2001).
3   Our emphasis.
4   That this is an imagined episode is readily given away by allowing the nurse enough time to sit down.
5   Kathy consciously refrains from talking, a clear signal that she is taking the time to listen.
6   Forgive us the technical language.
7   Though the vast majority of people say they want to die at home, most of them die in hospitals or nursing homes.

12 Nurses and stress

1 One proposed definition is that stress is anything that increases the secretion of glucocorticoids (Heurser and Lammers 2003).
2 "Generation Xers see their predecessors as self-indulgent, incompetent, morally bankrupt, and ruthlessly exploitative of the weak. Baby Boomers portray their young detractors as shiftless slackers unwilling to pay their dues and as rebels who expect free rides to the good life." We quote from the paper because of the graphic language though we do not know how widespread this problem may be.
3 An example of assertiveness reducing stress.
4 We think "emotional contagion" is an unfelicitous phrase since emotions evolved so as to evoke emotions in others and it is natural to experience to some degree the emotions of other. Perhaps "empathic overload", or "empathic excess" would work.
5 It remains to be seen if computers will free up nurses to be with their patients (Currell and Urquhart 2003).

13 Getting psychiatric consultation

1 To reduce wordiness the term 'psychiatric consultant' will replace 'psychiatic nurse or psychiatrist' unless a distinction between them must be made.
2 Some physicians, however, may be less satisfied with the results of referral of their outpatients to a psychiatrist (Brown and Weston 1992).
3 Methadone is usually ordered on a routinely scheduled basis but this patient may have eventually needed a chronic narcotic regimen.
4 The CDMHP in the state of Washington has the authority for involuntary psychiatric commitment of patients who, on the basis of a mental disorder, are a threat to themselves or others, or are gravely disabled.
5 The American term for old age psychiatrist is geriatric psychiatrist.
6 This scenario is so common that the experienced consultation/liaison psychiatrist can make the diagnosis by history alone.

Index